DATE DUE		
NOV 0 4 1996 S		
MAY 0 9 1997 S		
NOV 1 9 1997 S		

E.COLI O157

E.COLI O157

THE TRUE STORY OF A MOTHER'S BATTLE WITH A KILLER MICROBE

MARY HEERSINK

New Horizon Press   Far Hills, NJ

Requests for permission should be addressed to:
New Horizon Press
P.O. Box 669
Far Hills, NJ 07931

Heersink, Mary
        E. coli O157: The True Story of a Mother's Battle With a Killer Microbe.

Library of Congress Catalog Card Number: 96-68927

ISBN: 0-88282-143-1

New Horizon Press

Manufactured in the U.S.A.

2000 1999 1998 1997 1996 / 5 4 3 2 1

This book is dedicated to the following:

Riley Detwiler	1992-1993
Alexander Thomas Donley	1987-1993
Paige Hall	1993-1995
Scott Michael Hinkley	1990-1993
Lois Joy Galler	1989-1992
Eric Jackson Mueller	1980-1993
Michael James Nole	1991-1993
Katie O'Connell	1990-1992
Lauren Beth Rudolph	1986-1992
Kevin Allen Scott	1990-1994
Celina Schribbs	1992-1993
Jonathon Stephen Vassilowitch	1989-1992
Kristel Love	1980-1987

Contents

Acknowledgments

Focusing attention on a new and virulent microbe that overlaps into politics, public health, and corporate might has been a daunting task. The disillusionment I've encountered is only counterbalanced by the inspirational people who have impacted on this work, and this book. My gratitude to all these people working in the trenches to protect us all.

To:

Dr. Patricia Griffin, head of the Centers for Disease Control's Enteric Diseases for the cover's electronmicrograph of Escherichia coli O157:H7, and for her pioneering research on this pathogen and efforts to knit together a national surveillance net despite extreme underfunding.

Jof Goebbels, Willem Edel, and Enne de Boer of the Dutch Ministry of Health's Meat Inspectorate, who opened up their system to me, a system that proves it is possible to have a proper government response to O157:H7's public health hazard.

Carol Tucker Foreman of Safe Table Coalition, Caroline Smith de Waal of Center for Science in the Public Interest, Elaine Dodge of Government Accountability Project, and Donna Rosenbaum of Safe Tables Our Priority who have all worked tirelessly to reform irresponsible policy and to amplify the voices of victims.

Steve Cockerham, who exemplifies the federal meat inspectors brave enough to blow the whistle on the dangers of deregulative programs and sanitation violations in packing plants.

Steve Bjerklie for his encouraging feedback and friendship, as well as the groundbreaking work he did as editor of *Meat and*

Poultry magazine, holding a mirror up to his industry and casting a scorching light on its culpability in America's O157:H7 epidemic.

Craig Wilson of Frigoscandia, who in response to the human and economic costs of O157:H7, developed steam pasteurization, handing to industry the first truly effective tool for reducing pathogens, and who graciously included victims in every step of its verification and approval processes.

But most of all, to those left in the wreckage of this unforgiving microbe, who nonetheless found the fortitude to sound the alarm and fight for the safety of others: Nancy Donley, Kathy Allen, Jan Sowerby, Roni Rudolph, Rainer Mueller, Mike and Diana Nole, Laura and Darlene Day, Suzanne Kiner, Art O'Connell, Holly Scott, Bonnie Rock, Sonja Fendorf, Fred and Analese Thompson, Joe and Dorothy Dolan. It would have been so much easier to retreat into their private grief and pain.

And finally to my agent Bill Adler who knows firsthand the damage of pathogens in food and who encouraged me in this attempt to put a face on our nation's bacterial food borne illness crisis; Dennis McCarthy at New Horizon Press for his patience; and to my editor Joan Dunphy for expertly distilling my manuscript down to its essential story.

Author's Note

This book is based on my experiences, and reflects my perceptions of the past, present and future. The personalities, events, actions and conversations portrayed within the story have been reconstructed from my memory, hospital records, letters, personal papers, and press accounts. Some names and events have been altered to protect the privacy of individuals. Events involving the characters happened as described; only minor details have been altered.

1

How It Was

EVERYTHING WAS GOOD. Everything worked.

This was our world view. We were husband and wife. In the dark we'd hold each other, and our comfortable philosophy, close to our hearts. In a quieted house, we'd embrace it, marvel at it, make wishes we'd never have to revise it.

Both of us had been blessed from birth with good things. Everything was in place, immutable. We could not have engineered more perfect lives. We were grateful to our fate, our backgrounds, our education and our genetics for all that life provided.

Four children slept in upstairs bedrooms. Like all children are meant to, they slept blanketed in the security that they would wake up to love. Healthy blood pumped in their vessels. In their bodies, complex well-functioning processes continued all night as they turned and dreamt and grew.

It was how it always was.

It was how it always would be.

Everything worked. Everything was good.

Warm February days are not uncommon in Alabama. But that February had a strange unsettling feeling, an unnatural quality, to it. For one thing, our home was tainted by a rare disagreement between my husband and me. Something compelled him sixteen years after medical school to decide to study for the Florida medical boards. We argued often about it. All of my arguments made sense to me: all of his intensely private thoughts made sense to him.

"You've been in practice in Alabama for twelve years," I pointed out. "You love it here. You don't plan to move. You already have medical licenses in eighteen other states. Why are you collecting licenses like some people collect bumper stickers from national parks? You even keep your Canadian license, and God knows you're not going to practice there. You know your practice here is more complex and successful and busier than you can possibly handle, so what exactly is the point?"

Marnix, his brown hair tousled, his blue eyes fixed firmly on the patient's folder before him, didn't look up, which meant to me that he wasn't listening. I hated it when he hunkered down, waiting for my arguments to blow over. I hated it when he took cover under whatever he happened to be doing.

"Can you please put down that chart for one minute so you can hear me? And, Mila," I said to our daughter who had just sidled into the room, "out! Don't come in here. Dad and I aren't finished talking yet. I told you I'd be up to say good night in five minutes. Hop on up. Now."

At seven, Mila was uncannily drawn to private conversations between her dad and me. She was very precocious and wanted to observe how to be even more mature than she was. What better way than to sneak in on her parents' disagreements?

"Where were we?" I said to Marnix after Mila left. "You know how happy you were when you finished your fellowship and passed the ophthalmology boards. You told me you were so glad that you'd never have to study for another exam again. Remember you told me you were so happy that you had dreams about it? So why are you killing yourself for something you don't need and will never use?"

He didn't have a decent counter argument. Even more maddening, he didn't try to defend his plan. It inflamed me more that I couldn't engage him. "Marnix, it's getting really hard. You're gone so long, and it's every week. I hate being alone all night. The kids are too much for me to do all by myself for five days at a time. When you studied at medical school, we didn't have children to consider. This is just getting to be brutal. I'm so angry at you. I can't understand why you're doing this."

But I did understand. I had learned to recognize this character flaw in my husband: unmitigated ambition. He must always be improving, carving out new territory, developing big projects. He was good at it, and we owed our freedom and comfort to it. But often he couldn't turn off his ambition long enough to enjoy what he had accomplished.

I blamed it on his being Dutch. Do you think the Dutch can accept the boundaries that the North Sea imposes on their land? Hell no, they push the ocean back with a brilliant system of canals and windmills, dikes and confidence. It's a national affliction, this over ambition. My nagging was useless against centuries of collective determination.

So every Wednesday afternoon, Marnix drove 200 miles to Birmingham to study at the University of Alabama medical complex until Sunday evening. There he followed a review course that would prepare him for the Florida examination which would be given the first week of March. He described this exam as a sort of floodgate intended to hold back the overflow of physicians who wanted to work part-time when they retired to the Sunshine State. Other states had issued him licenses through reciprocity: Florida required that he prove himself all over again.

He was into marathon studying. All the basic science he had forgotten had to be relearned, and he had to catch up on new developments that had occurred in the last sixteen years. He holed up in the university library, cramming information in the fields of hematology, pediatrics, nephrology—all the disciplines, in my opinion, that a forty-one-year-old, sub-specialized, fellowship-trained eye surgeon would never ever need.

FEBRUARY 19

Our youngest son, Bayne, was turning nine this weekend, and not only would my husband miss his third son's birthday, but he hadn't even seen the new tree house yet. It had been two weeks since a friend and I built this big birthday present in the woods. Marnix wasn't going to be here for the unveiling, nor for the party at which the little boys would break it in, nor for the installation of the finishing touches: a pulley system, a flagpole and spy holes. He didn't even know what it looked like, or where in the woods it was built.

2

Incubation

It was only the last weekend of February, yet it felt as warm as April. I went about my duties, pushing my irritation at Marnix to the back of my mind. Damion was going on a campout with the Scouts. He wouldn't need the winter sleeping bag we'd bought. But he could sleep on top of it, I thought as I pulled into the parking lot where the boys were gathering. Most of the Scouts were here already. Leaders were talking to moms, some boys were throwing a football, and others were loading the groceries into the rear of the church bus. I pulled our van up to this controlled confusion, to thank John Holan, Damion's scout leader, while Damion bolted out of the van to join his buddies.

John was a great guy. He was a man's man who loved the outdoors, and he actually seemed to enjoy taking his troop of preadolescents into the woods each month. Damion looked forward to these campouts, which surprised us because he was never big on discomfort. But he always came back happy and filthy and feeling good about all the mysterious things boys get out of living primitively with other guys.

The merit badge they'd earn this weekend was in "food preparation." To earn it, the boys would plan, purchase, and cook all the meals themselves.

"Hey, John," I said, "Damion's got the hamburger buns here. Do you want him to set them on top of the bags?"

A small voice said to me: Bags? Don't the Scouts have coolers? I couldn't remember. But there must be coolers, I thought vaguely: the boys had bought hamburger meat to cook tomorrow night.

Coolers would be needed to keep the meat cold in this warm weather. I felt a slight jarring, a concern so small, yet big enough to form a question for the leaders.

"Do you have coolers?" The question must have been answered to my satisfaction. I don't remember. I must have been reassured, because the image of raw meat stored in grocery bags did not stir again.

Evil comes into our lives in such seemingly inconsequential, innocuous ways. Perhaps we see an element of it, a shiny small out-of-place detail that glistens precipitously, some little fragment of glass, rippled maybe, or faceted, distorted only enough to flash the slightest warning. But we shield our eyes from its glint. We justify. We trust. We back away from the little signal. And so the silent fracturing begins unnoticed.

I left Damion there healthy and strong and seemingly invulnerable in the humid parking lot. I smiled as the church bus drove away, a bus loaded with boisterous Boy Scouts and bags filled with groceries highlighted in the back window. Can you think of a more innocuous, innocent sight? I thought, and then promptly forgot it, immersed in our busy life.

FEBRUARY 22 THROUGH FEBRUARY 29

This was the week in between, the week the evil was working.

I had forgiven Marnix for his absence. After all, his examination was only days away, on March 3. This Florida bitterness would, I thought, soon fade into an old argument I wouldn't be able to remember and we'd get to have him home on weekends again.

During the week, Bayne spray painted the tree house with streaks of camouflage. Damion emerged from his camping weekend contented and properly dirty. He'd loved every minute of it. Sebastian was going to his teachers and gathering schoolwork that he would miss the following week. On Saturday, he, Damion and I would travel to Florida in the van. Sebastian would spend a week at tennis camp, and Damion would be at space camp for the week.

That meant the younger children, Bayne and Mila, would be left at home with a baby-sitter. Mila was very mindful of the amount of time I spent with her. If it was not an exclusive time, it didn't count. Mila needed my complete attention once in a while, but rarely got it. This week I had promised that we'd have an afternoon together to do whatever she wanted. We'd forget about the boys' lessons and their schedule of games. We'd be just us two.

All of the children felt the imbalance of time and attention in our large family. This season we were focused on ten-year-old Sebastian who frequently needed to be taken to tennis tournaments on weekends and who had daily practices that chopped up the afternoons for all of us. The other children got left behind while I chauffeured our tennis player, or else had to go along for the ride. Mila was the only one to articulate the beginnings of resentment. She was sharp and insightful. And outspoken. She demanded what was rightfully hers, as she must in a family with three older brothers. And what she demanded now was attention. This demand was more compelling than usual because she and Bayne were to be left with the sitter all next week. When you are seven, seven days without your parents is a long time. I was sorry she'd be without me for so long, but when we got back from Florida, I promised her, I'd make up for it.

This was one of the subsets of our belief system: everything worked, but if it was ever temporarily out of balance, it could be righted. We were, after all, engineers of our own fate. Right?

FRIDAY, FEBRUARY 28

I stood in Damion's bedroom and told him, "All right, this is the deal. Tomorrow morning you have the soccer tournament, and in the afternoon we go to Florida. You can spend tonight at Matt Hall's if you promise to go to bed early and if you will quietly let yourself out in the morning and not disturb everyone."

"Okay, Mom."

"I'll be by at seven-thirty. You be up and ready to go to your game. And try not to wake up anyone else. Okay, D.?"

"Okay, Mom."

I smiled at him, hardly noticing anything amiss. "Don't forget," I said. "Gather all your games and clothes and soccer gear. Be up and ready by the time I get there."

3

Lightening

At his friend Matt's house the next morning, Damion, always a dutiful child, was ready. He always wanted to do the right thing. Whatever we asked was okay. A typical firstborn, he wanted to please, be compliant. Today as usual he was doing the right thing, sitting at the Halls' kitchen table waiting for me. But something about him wasn't right. As I entered the courtyard and approached the French doors, I could see it. He was hunched over the table, head resting on one arm, his long languid body in a slouch. Opening the door, I saw that his face was as pale as the whitewashed cabinets of our friends' pristine kitchen.

I thought, That's strange, he never sits like that. "Hey, pup, what's up?" I called. "Did you get to sleep too late? What's the matter, D.? You don't look too fired up for the tournament. Thanks for being ready, though."

Karen Hall, Matt's mother, came into the kitchen in her blue bathrobe, saying, "I'm really sorry he's sick."

Then Damion told me he'd been up all night with cramps and diarrhea but he had tried not to wake Matt's parents.

"I gave him some Tylenol in the middle of the night," Karen told me. "It's probably just a quick bug," she said to Damion, "or maybe the pizza last night didn't agree with you."

"Thanks," I said with that conspiratorial nod which for mothers is the high five sign. I turned to my son. "Well, let's go, D. I got you a croissanwich for breakfast, and it's in the van with your jersey."

As I walked him to the car, I was giving him the once-over as my mind flitted about. Damion was never sick. This was just what

7

we didn't need on a day when we were trying to get out of town after a soccer tournament. We threaded our way through the Halls' sunny courtyard. Damion seemed light, thin, luminous. Always so tall and thin, he looked lighter to me. It wasn't only a blanching of his complexion, though he was pale. There was another kind of diminishing somehow. If a doctor looked at him, he'd probably remark, "A little washed out from lack of sleep. Maybe he has a touch of virus." If we were to put him on the doctor's scale, he'd probably show only a pound or two of weight loss. The diarrhea would account for that. No, what I detected was not a lightness that could be measured. There was a lightening in his walk, his replies, his alertness. I sensed it, but I did not allow myself to see.

Something was fading about him. A distance was being established, as if perspective and space made him recede a bit. Not a lot, just a tone lighter, not enough to consider on such a busy day.

We drove away in the van and came to Bruno's market where I often shopped. "Well," I said, "let's get something for your diarrhea. And some Gatorade for your games. I'll be right back, D."

It took only a few minutes in the express line at Bruno's to purchase Emetrol, Pepto-Bismol, and lemon-lime Gatorade. Quickly I got back in the car. "This'll fix it, honey. Take these two tablets, D." Then I looked at him again. "I can't believe you've put on only one shin guard in the time I was shopping. Can you please sit up and finish getting ready? Come on, bud, we're almost to Westgate."

When I parked at the Westgate Park soccer field, I saw through the windshield the boys and coaches. In the rear view mirror, bright sunshine dazzled. "D., will you please sit up? Okay, look. I'll tell Coach McLean you're out for the first game. Would you please start drinking some of this Gatorade? If you can't eat any of your croissant, at least drink some fluids so we can get you in shape for your noon game. Come on, boy."

Striding over to the huddle of the Dothan Shockers, I felt badly that Damion would miss the game and possibly the whole Azalea Dogwood tournament. Not that he was an exceptional goalie, but duty to one's team is a lesson we tried to impart to the children. Damion's long arm span allowed him to be an effective goalie, and his laid-back temperament was up to the pressure of the position. And he loved it. Sebastian usually outshone him in sports and had an impressive collection of trophies and accolades. Soccer was a game in which Damion didn't have to compete with his younger brother. Being a member of Dothan's spring traveling soccer team was all his. The weekend travel to tournaments was his opportunity for camaraderie. He was making diverse friends and developing sportsmanship. And he was doing something we sensed was very important to our oldest child, developing confidence in himself.

Coach McLean walked over to our van to commiserate with Damion that he would not be able to play this morning.

As the soccer match began, I drove home and put Damion to bed. "Just for a few hours," I said in answer to his weak protests. However, what was supposed to be a nap turned into an entire day in bed. Damion got up only to use the bathroom. I gave him Tylenol and Emetrol each time.

Growing up in a large family with a father who was a doctor, and then marrying a physician, I had developed a nonchalance toward these little illnesses. One of my earliest memories is of my brother being diagnosed with scarlet fever during a family vacation in Maine. He didn't seem very sick to us children, but my parents spoke about the disease as if it were a serious threat. My father hurried back from his trip into town, lined all eleven of us up around the kitchen table, and gave us shots. This, he told us, would make us safe. We were magically shielded. Medicine built a membrane around our world that disease couldn't penetrate. I still believed it.

In Marnix's and my family, we'd easily dealt with childhood illnesses. Our four children had suffered their share of ear infections, chicken pox, croup—all the nuisance sicknesses that made life seem like a television sitcom. They were problems so easy to resolve. Earache? Go to our cabinet, pull out the antibiotic. Out of Amoxil? Have Papa call in a prescription to the pharmacy and ten minutes later it's being delivered. I rarely had to enter the bureaucracy of the health care system and never had to wait in the crowded reception room of an overworked pediatrician, hoping my child would not spread his infection or pick up someone else's. If one of the children became sick, Marnix was always there to dismiss its importance. "That's good," he'd tell me when I told him Sebastian or Bayne had a fever or diarrhea. "Think of it as a good thing, Mary. He needs to build up resistance. He needs to be exposed to a little dirt. If the children don't go through these bugs, they cannot build up proper immune systems."

And so, all the normal childhood illnesses scrolled across the screen of the years like tiny blips on four robust lines. Marnix was there to interpret, prescribe, reassure. But this Saturday he was out of town.

Of course he called, renewing his objections to our going to Florida. His objections were more concerned with my driving at night and the duration of the trip. I brushed them aside. Neither of us felt serious concern about Damion when I described his symptoms.

However, Fred Ernst called. He had seen us at the soccer field. Fred was a physician, family friend, and a father whom we saw at many of our children's sporting events. "Mary," he said, "I can go get you something from the hospital pharmacy if you need it. I know that Marnix is out of town and most pharmacies are closed for the weekend, is there anything you need?"

I told him that I couldn't think of anything other than letting Damion rest before taking the trip. I described what over-the-counter medicines I was giving Damion. Fred was against my leaving town with him.

"He was very lethargic when I saw him in your van, Mary. He looked septic to me. You don't need to be traveling with him when he feels this badly. At the very least, you should be alert for certain symptoms." He went on to tell me to look for high temperature spikes and bleeding. His reaction seemed a little extreme to me, and I basically disregarded his sense of alarm.

"It's only a little bug, Fred," I said. "When you have a large family like ours, someone is always coming down with something."

Fred's voice over the phone remained worried. "You must call me if you notice a change or need anything. Maureen and I will be home after Ryan's next game."

Thanking Fred for his concern, I dismissed his words as simply a friendly if anxious gesture.

Yet, when I woke Damion hours later, he could not shake off his grogginess. "Damion, can you stay awake just a minute?" I pleaded. "I think you really should drink some Gatorade. If you don't take fluids, you could get dehydrated. Come on, D.D., you really need to drink. If you want to get better in time for space camp, we've got to get that belly settled."

What was going on? He couldn't drink. He couldn't eat. When he wasn't in the bathroom, he was in bed in a deep sleep—a far away sleep, hard to call him back from. Receding. Was he receding from us? It was then I began to think about what Fred had said. I pushed the thoughts away. No. I was being silly. I was becoming an overprotective mother.

At this point I made the subconscious decision to do the unreasonable: to leave for the trip anyway. An internal, irrational process.

"Come on, D. Get up. Let's go."

SATURDAY AFTERNOON

Silver sunlight was fading, afternoon was ending, and the van, loaded with Damion's clothes for space camp and Sebastian's gear for tennis camp, stood dark and bulging. In the back were blankets, the Gatorade, the ineffective medicines, towels and a large cooking pot in case Damion needed to vomit. I squeezed in the last suitcases and recited instructions to our baby-sitter, Liz.

Damion drifted away from his brothers and sister, walking slowly toward the van, looking strangely aloof. Increasingly, this aura about him disturbed me. I searched for words to describe to myself what it was about him that bothered me. A lightening, somehow. A *lightness* that couldn't be measured or explained by lost body fluids or pale skin. A lightening of the person that couldn't be accurately described, a lightening to his movements, diffuse replies, diminishing alertness, a distance being established.

Now it's clear to me: he was starting to leave us.

Now I see it. At the time, I only felt the gathering compulsion within me to get my son out of our small town as if going away would somehow help him. I tried to tell myself I was imagining the changes I saw. I made myself refocus on our leave-taking.

"Liz, tell Marnix we'll be okay. I know he doesn't want us to go, but tell him I decided it was the best thing to do."

I turned to the two towheaded children standing before me.

"Bye bye, angels. You be very good for Liz. I'll see you guys in one short week. D., climb in the back there with the blankets."

As the car pulled away, I glanced in the rearview mirror. The children and Liz were waving. I shifted the mirror slightly to see the back seat. The last glint of daylight fired up the outline of Damion's face against the window like streaks of lightning edging a cloud before the thunderbolt strikes.

SATURDAY EVENING

Driving slowly, I made the appropriate turns and in a short while we were on the highway. Once the measured monotony of driving was well established, I began to question myself. Is this the smart thing to do? Starting out on a seven-hour drive at sundown when I was already tired and one of my children was sick in the back? Marnix had warned on the phone from Birmingham that it wasn't wise to do this. He didn't like me driving long stretches at night, ever. Fred Ernst had told me it was not a good idea to let Damion travel. Why hadn't I waited until tomorrow morning when I could drive in daylight and Damion would surely be better? With such seemingly impulsive decisions, when we allow instinct to override logic and reality, we seed the future.

SATURDAY NIGHT

Pines curtained in parasitic Spanish moss, Cenozoic cypress and mimosa, stretches of shallow swamp glint past the car. Northwest Florida is a dark place, the darkest I've ever seen. Driving from Marianna to Lake City, 170 miles east along Route 10, the dark was interrupted only by the distant dome of light that was Tallahassee. It was a darkness as heavy as the limbs on the live oaks by the side of the road.

Northwest Florida's darkness is blackened by the eons, encrusted with continuity. If, while driving along, I eliminated the center strip of the road from view, this black and heavy landscape became again what it once was: ancient, primordial. I cracked my window to stay awake on the cool damp exhalation of black-green leaves, black soil, and green-black creatures.

My headlights intruded on the landscape. They illuminated a path through the old forms that loomed and then receded, loomed

My headlights intruded on the landscape. They illuminated a path through the old forms that loomed and then receded, loomed and receded until we reached civilization again at I-75 South. Three fragile people encased in steel racing along at seventy miles an hour.

It was quiet, too. Turning on the interior lights, I checked on the sleeping boys. Sebastian slept in the passenger seat beside me, his healthy preadolescent body scrunched up on the seat, his pink face pressed against the fogged window. In the rearview mirror Damion was curled away from me. I could not see him clearly but he felt my glance and stirred.

"Mom," he said, "I have to go again."

Fortunately, the next rest stop was not that far. Soon I pulled the van in and kept the motor running while he used the bathroom. I could only find country music on the radio. I knew from experience this would be the only listening choice for hours until we got to the college town of Gainesville. In the parking lot of one of America's generic rest stops, I thought about why country music was so popular. Much of America is still big, expansive, and lonely. Some of its people are out on dark roads in monstrous trucks. Many of them wander around forsaken places like this at night. Country music fills the void, the large emptiness, with emotion. Love, loneliness, lust, cuckoldry, crying in dark, musty bars. The point of country music is to keep us from feeling so small, to give a certain sense of scale. That was what I was thinking as Damion returned from the bathroom. Country music was about the immensity of human emotion.

"Come on, pup. I want to get at least to Ocala tonight."

Damion weakly slid the van door shut. It didn't close tightly, so he had to do it again.

"You okay, D.?" I whispered so that Sebastian wouldn't awaken. "Is it getting any better? Less diarrhea now?"

His voice was thin, miserable. "No. Um. I'm sorry, Mom, I couldn't help it. My pants got dirty."

"That's all right, baby. We'll get you cleaned up later."

Realizing that I'd better find a place to stay, clean Damion up and assess his condition, I decided against going all the way to Ocala and opted for Gainesville, only ninety minutes away. I was disappointed I couldn't do the whole seven hours that night. I wanted the trip to be over. I'd have to scale back. We'll have lots of choices of hotels in Gainesville, I told myself optimistically.

Not true. We drove around the town in frustration, trying first one motel, then another: Econo Lodge, Holiday Inn, La Quinta, Hampton Inn. All filled. We became more and more discouraged. Sebastian ran into each lobby to inquire at the desk while Damion, my sweater wrapped around his waist, discreetly used the bathroom. There was a bikers' convention in town, and all the rooms from Gainesville south were booked by middle-aged motorcyclists in leather, on their way to reenact their youth in Daytona.

Finally, at one in the morning, I pleaded with the orange-haired woman behind the Hilton registration desk. "Please," I told her, "my son is sick, and I don't think we can make it to Ocala." She handed over the key to the last room. How strange, I thought. Us and the Hell's Angels at the Hilton.

Encouraging Damion to get into the shower, I felt almost satisfied. After all, I had gotten most of the drive accomplished, and I'd found a nice room in the crowded town. Those must be good signs. "Now let's get some rest," I called to the boys.

But our sleep was disturbed by Damion's frequent trips to the bathroom. In one of my unsettling dreams, he didn't walk past my bed to the bathroom, but floated luminously in the dark toward the hallway door.

Running after him into the parking lot in my dream, my foot caught in the spokes of a bike. As metal crashed on pavement, my eyes flew open to see the hotel room, flooded by morning.

The sound of people's voices calling to each other and closing car doors outside our ground floor window made me realize the nightmarish crashing had really only been a trunk slamming shut.

4

Roller Coaster Pass

I must have dozed off again. When I awoke, I couldn't believe the clock read ten-thirty. "How could we possibly have slept till ten-thirty? I've got to get these boys moving," I said, spurring myself on. Damion was reluctant to get out of bed, but I knew I had to get them up and dressed while the dining room was still open for breakfast. Damion hadn't eaten anything in thirty-six hours. A big breakfast would help him get going. Then, I thought, a couple more hours to Tampa we'd get Sebastian into tennis camp well before the orientation at four. I'd worry about getting Damion to the space camp at Cape Canaveral on the east coast later. He looked worse this morning, so we'd probably have to nurse him along another day or so before he could join his group. Damion had attended space camp in Huntsville, Alabama twice before. And although the layout of the camp in Titusville, Florida was different, the program was the same. I was not concerned about him missing the beginning. Before checking out of the hotel, I called the officials at the space camp to tell them Damion was down with the flu. "I'll keep him out the first day," I explained.

"No problem," said the camp director. "Just bring him when he feels better."

At breakfast Damion would not eat anything. What was more worrisome was that he wouldn't take even one sip of his juice. "Damion, when was the last time you drank some liquid?" I asked.

He stared off into space. "Yesterday in Bruno's parking lot."

That began a tug of war. For the next two hours on the drive to Tampa I pleaded with him to drink some Gatorade from the bottle between us in the front seats. "Come on, D. You've lost a lot of fluids. You've got to be thirsty by now." But he refused, as though I was asking the utterly impossible.

"Damion, are you peeing?"

"Uh-huh."

"Good. Are you having as much diarrhea as before? I mean, I know you have to use the bathroom a lot, but do you think it's mostly out of your system by now?"

"Um."

"What's that mean? Is it more or less? Come on, D. Can you stay awake a little while and help me find the Zephyr Hills exit. We ought to be there soon."

"Okay," he said in a lackluster voice.

"D., as I was asking, more diarrhea today, or less?"

"Well, it's a little more since it turned red."

"Damn it!" I said, not quietly enough.

Now the road felt like a trap, a long greasy trap from which I'd better find the right exit. Damion continued not to drink, he was pale, he couldn't stay awake, and there was blood in his stool. I reviewed his symptoms as I drove the last ten minutes of highway. It wasn't long before I pulled the van up to the guardhouse of the Saddlebrook Tennis and Golf Resort. I resolved to keep a positive attitude.

"Sebastian, look how beautiful a place this is! Jennifer Capriati lives in one of these houses." Beautifully landscaped brick and stucco homes were set back on winding streets. There were more joggers and bicyclists than automobiles. Passing a tennis complex, swimming pools and condominiums, we wound our way to the registration area. I decided we would spend the night here. Disregarding the beauty around us, I planned the order of phone calls I would make in a few minutes.

As Sebastian and I checked in, Damion headed for the bathroom again. When he returned, his eyes looked sunken in. "No." He shook his head. He didn't have the energy to investigate the pools and cafes with his brother. Not able to find an empty chair, he leaned against the cool limestone wall.

Yes, I told myself, we needed to spend the night right here, and I needed to get on the phone. Damion's lips were becoming cracked. He had won the battle of not drinking the Gatorade.

"How many keys?" the blond receptionist asked in a singsong voice.

"Two please. Can the children use these to charge food? Yes, he's already been registered by mail at Hopman's Camp. Last thing," I said to the receptionist, "do you know anything about nearby hospitals? That lady there? Thank you."

The polite receptionist referred me to a woman behind an information desk across the lobby. But a very loud and huge German woman was arguing with her about limousine service to the airport. So I went to find Sebastian outside. When I returned with him, the argument was continuing. Now the angry woman was fortified in her argument by her even more irritated short, plump husband arguing in the classic Teutonic manner. The man was red faced and agitated. I looked around for Damion. Pale and listless, he was still leaning against the wall.

"Come on, baby," I said. "Let's go to the room and get you comfortable. You can lie down while I get Sebastian settled into his program."

While Sebastian unpacked the car for us, I used the room phone and tried to call Marnix at his hotel in Birmingham. There was no answer. I glanced at my watch. It was mid-afternoon; he would still be at the library. I'd have to wait until that night to tell him about Damion and ask what to do.

Next, I made a quick call to the Halls' house. "Hey, Matt. Damion's mom here. Is your mom there? Oh, when will they be back? Listen, Matt, honey. Is anyone at your house sick? No one got sick after the pizza Friday night? You're sure no one has an upset stomach? Oh well, Matt, thank you. Damion's okay. He just feels cruddy. Say hi to your mom for me."

While Sebastian alternated carrying a handful of things from the van with flipping through the television channels to see what kind of entertainment the room promised, I made another telephone call. It was to the nurse on duty for Dr. Forston, our pediatrician back home. "Hello, Debbie. This is Mary Heersink. I'm calling from Florida. I'm sorry to interrupt your Sunday, but I'm getting concerned about our Damion." I described his symptoms.

She patiently listened, then questioned me about his temperature, the diarrhea, his lethargy, the blood he mentioned. Just as I was feeling sorry to have bothered her for something that didn't sound so worrisome, she advised me, "With blood in the stool, it's important to get him checked. Maybe you can get some medication at an emergency room to make him comfortable."

I love our pediatricians and am always grateful to their devoted staff. It was a relief to speak with Debbie and get her opinion that Damion's condition probably warranted a quick check.

While I was on the phone, Sebastian had returned to the room again. Now I turned to him, trying to sound calm and collected. "Sebastian, hurry. Let's get you to your orientation meeting. While you're there, I'll rent a bike for you to get around on."

Then I spoke to Damion. "D.D., we'll be back in thirty minutes. Can you jump into the shower while I'm gone? I'll pick up a Sprite for you while I'm out. Once I get this tennis business out of the way, we'll run into town to find some medicine at the hospital. Okay? Just put on some clean clothes after your shower. Be right back."

We left Damion lying on the bed, promising to be ready by the time we returned.

When we came back forty minutes later, the room was darkened. Damion was asleep again. On the bathroom floor were dirty clothes. Watery red-brown stains were on his underwear. The shower curtain dripped water onto the floor. Pushing the curtain back into the tub, I saw a long clot of bloody mucus that had not slid down the drain.

"Oh, man," I said.

The emergency room looked like a battle zone. The large gray-haired receptionist behind the metal desk told me, "First, you'll have to wait for a triage nurse." A little later, I described Damion's symptoms to that nurse at her battered desk.

"Right," she said, not looking up from the form she was filling in.

Obviously, I was boring her, but now that we were here I was determined to make her listen.

"And, ma'am, also, I think there is blood in his stool."

She looked weary. "Well, it's going to be a while. It's very busy this afternoon with emergencies. We'll call you when the doctor can see him."

My forehead scrunched. Okay, I know I don't belong here, I said to her silently. I'm traveling. I should just get my husband to call in a prescription. I don't want to be here either, lady, but now I'm stuck, I thought, watching her.

Aloud I said nothing.

We went back to the linoleum-floored casualty room. The sitcom *Head of the Class* blared over our heads, sick people clustered about. Most were dirty and pathetic looking. Normally, Damion would have been nudging me and saying, Look, Mom. Watch this guy. He's funny. Do you like this show, Mom? Instead, he rested his head on my lap and said not a word. Sometimes we'd have three chairs across. Other times the room filled up with more wounded, and he'd have to sit up and lean against me. Along with the annoying television, a loud clock ticked the evening away.

At eight o'clock, I called Sebastian at the resort. "Bombie, look. I know I said we'd be back in an hour and a half, but we're still waiting to get some medicine for D. Did you get enough to eat from room service? Look, you need to turn the television off and get to sleep. You're in a safe place so just lock the deadbolt and don't answer the door. My key will open it when we get in later. I'll call the front desk and tell them to check you. Here's the hospital number. Tell them I'm in the emergency room if you need me."

I felt awful leaving Sebastian so long alone, but at least Saddlebrook Resort was a closed, secure community. "Brush your teeth and then lights out, bomber. Damion and I will sneak back in as soon as we can. Nighty night, baby."

Next, I dialed Marnix's hotel. "Hi, dear. I don't want you to worry, but I've got Damion waiting in an E.R. here. I want a doctor to check on his diarrhea. It has become bloody. And all he does is sleep. Let's see, it's called Lennox Hospital, and it's on the north edge of Tampa, about twenty-five minutes from Saddlebrook. No, no idea what kind of reputation it has. I pulled in when I saw it was a large building. It seemed like it would be okay. Look, I know it's no big deal, but Stan Forston's nurse told me it would be reasonable to get him checked out. You know, he won't drink anything, either. I doubt it. He hasn't had any more than a mouthful of food since

Friday evening. I *have*, Marnix. I told him I'd even *pay* him to drink. No, I don't know how soon he'll be seen. We got here at five. We are low priority with diarrhea."

I looked from the pay phone over to Damion across the room, his face like wax in the harsh light.

"You wouldn't believe this place. One man came in carrying his fingers in a kitchen towel. Another man is crying about his leg. And the children are ragged and dirty. One witch of a mother keeps telling her barefooted little girl that she will beat her if she gets out of her seat. There are a lot of people that look like migrant workers, in pitiful shape. You think I should just leave? Yep, you're right. Once you get in the system. . . . Now I see what you mean about staying out of hospitals if you possible can."

Marnix asked about Sebastian. "No, he's not here, and I'm glad he's not. He's fed and locked in our room, hopefully getting to sleep by now. Will you call him to say good night? It's room nine-o-five. Do you still have the Saddlebrook number I gave you? Yeah, that's it. I know, I know. I hate it that he is alone this long, too. I dashed over here for a doctor to take a quick look, but it hasn't worked out that way. Listen, I'm not going to call you any more tonight. I'm just going to get Damion medicine and get out of here. You may as well get some sleep. I will, I will. Look. I'm sure he's fine. I'll let you know the diagnosis in the morning. Thanks, dear. Love you, too."

Another quarter got me the Saddlebrook desk. They would have their security guard listen at our room door every hour or so to make sure everything was all right inside. They would not wake Sebastian.

At quarter after eleven, Damion was finally called to an examining room. A young nurse took his history and vital signs. As I gave her the details, she scrawled some notes. I told her about the fever, the lack of fluid intake, the blood I saw. Then she left us. We had nearly an hour of silence. Damion was soon sound asleep. I began to feel like a real idiot, waiting six hours to ask a question about simple diarrhea.

A doctor with a big, kind, bearded face, weary eyes, and a pony tail longer than mine, entered the cubicle. "I'm Dr. Marinelli," he said. He listened to Damion's chest, palpated his abdomen, and read over the nurse's chart. He didn't rush us or make me feel ridiculous to bother him about a routine gastrointestinal upset. He was careful and meticulous.

He said, "I'll see you again after we get the results on some blood work and the report from Radiology."

"Radiology?" I repeated, my voice trembling. I never expected that.

The waiting began again. Damion's stretcher was moved and parked in a lineup of gurneys outside the radiology department. From one of the stretchers a beefy motorcyclist with brown oily hair bragged to an older diabetic man about how many pins were in his legs from a lifetime of crashes. At the same time, the diabetic's wife swore to her husband that this time, if the hospital admitted him, she was not going to sneak him home. A middle-aged accident victim lifted his head to tell his wife to be sure to get the names of the doctors for the lawsuit. Damion dozed through this absurdity, and I wondered about the state of medicine in our litigious society. Defensive medicine, that was why we were in this long lineup. I also wondered if this emergency department had any chairs I could pull into the hall. There didn't appear to be any, so I remained standing.

Three hours later, Dr. Marinelli found us in another hallway. By then I was sitting on the floor beside the gurney's wheels. A nurse with him pushed an empty wheelchair.

"I'm admitting your son to the hospital, Mrs. Heersink," the doctor said.

"You're kidding," I responded stupidly. I was so very tired. As he talked about pending lab results, the edematous colon shown on the x-ray films, and the pediatrician he'd called in, Dr. Marinelli bent down to help me gather my belongings off the floor. "In what way did the large intestine not look right?" I asked, scrambling for my things.

The doctor shook his head. "We'll have to see," he said.

The nurse was helping Damion into the wheelchair. Red stained sheets were dragged off the gurney.

Dr. Marinelli glared at them. "No one told me about the blood!" he said angrily.

With unanswerable questions revolving in my mind, I followed the wheelchair to the room where Damion would stay. I tried to reassure him. Tired and weak, he fell asleep.

It was quarter after four in the morning.

Leaving the hospital, I found my car parked all alone in the lot, and drove towards the resort on a fog-filled road. I wanted to be in bed. At least Damion was settled and asleep in a private hospital room. The fog obscured everything. Barely able to see the line in the middle of the road, I slowed down to fifteen miles per hour. No other cars were on the road. Who else would be crawling through this fog, except someone in an emergency situation? I scanned the fog for signs of the intersection near Saddlebrook, particularly the Burger King. It was about a twenty-minute drive to the hospital on our way in. So where the heck was it now?

"God, I'm tired," I murmured. I'm so tired. Let me think. I have to think clearly about this. Okay, if I set the alarm for half past five, I'll have time to write Sebastian a note and to lay out his rackets and clothes. I'd better change my clothes, too. If this fog gets out of here, I can be back at the hospital by half past six.

Yes, I thought. That will be good. I wouldn't see Sebastian awake, but I knew that pediatricians did their rounds early, maybe seven o'clock or so. I wanted to be at the hospital by then. Yes, that was it, that was what I had to do.

5

Acceleration

THERE IS A NAME I'VE FORGOTTEN. If I tried very hard to remember it, I'm sure I could. Or I could look it up. It's in the records. It simply escapes me. That is a part of healing, I suppose. Marnix can't remember her name either, and I try to keep it repressed for both of us.

Even today we make a point of not talking about her. I know his feelings toward her. "Infuriating" is the word he used to describe her. Truly, I'm not angry with her. She just got dragged into a case that was way over her head. I'll call her "the Asian doctor."

What I can't forget was the day Damion became her patient. It started uneventfully. The Asian doctor strode purposefully and confidently into Damion's room while I was on the phone with Marnix. She was small and had her black hair in a tight bun and was smiling an inscrutable smile suitable for a CIA operative. "Mrs. Heersink," she said, "I'm quite positive everything is perfectly all right. We'll keep him on IV fluids a short while, just as a precautionary measure. I'm certain he will do beautifully. Yes, I'd be delighted to speak with your husband."

She spoke in short staccato bursts into the phone. "Yes, Dr. Heersink. Oh, yes, everything is fine here. Lab work? Yes, I will order another CBC. Yes, I can order a stool culture as well. Shigella, salmonella, campylobacter. Vibrio, too. Yes, all four. No, I'm quite confident everything will resolve itself in quick time. Yes, irritated colon. Yes, that can be perfectly common."

When the call concluded, I asked, "Doctor, what is the significance of blood in the stool?"

I felt like a bubble-headed housewife who had no right to ask medical questions. "Oh, just a little colitis, nothing to become alarmed about. These cases of diarrhea can be severe enough to irritate the bowel and cause a little blood in the stool. It's nothing we professionals worry about, dear. I will check back with you later in the day. Everything is in order. He is doing beautifully."

"Okay, Thank you for checking on him, doctor," I said softly.

EARLY AFTERNOON

Damion slept his day away. He had intermittent fever up to 103 degrees. This was consistent with the Asian doctor's feelings about the flu. I was grateful to see the fluids dripping into him from the IV, because, whenever he roused from sleep, he still refused to drink.

When they had first settled him into the room in the middle of the night, it had been awful for Damion. First, it was hard for him to relinquish his underwear. He undressed under the privacy of his open-in-the-back hospital gown and the sheets. I took those soiled pants back to our room at Saddlebrook and dropped them on the bathroom floor with the other ones. Nor had starting the IV been easy for Damion. He'd never been stuck with a needle other than for immunization. I could see he was distressed when the nurse inserted the needle into the back of his left hand.

By this morning he had already felt the indignities of being prodded, stuck with needles, and x-rayed in the emergency room. All difficult issues of privacy for an eleven-year-old. These indecencies didn't disturb him now. He slept and slept. I watched him and repeated to myself my old mantra. Everything was going to be fine. Everything was good. I exhaustedly stretched out on the chair-bed contraption in the corner.

Damion woke to use the bathroom again. When he came out pushing his IV pole in a clumsy manner, he said sleepily, "Mom, it's getting worse."

I looked into the bathroom to see what he meant. It was shocking. It was as though someone had poured a gallon of clotted blood into the toilet. "Leave it, D. Let's not flush it so the nurse can see it." He was too weak to protest this additional indignity. This had to be more than an irritated colon, more than "just a little colitis."

E.COLI O157

Asking the nurse to look at it got no reaction. In fact, I began to notice that the nursing staff seemed mostly absent from the room. They came in once every three hours to record Damion's vital signs but that was all. When I telephoned my sister Grace in Connecticut who has a nursing background, she was surprised to hear that Damion was on IV fluids without having urine output measured.

Grace asked if I felt the medical staff knew what they were doing. She offered to call a family friend who practiced pediatric ophthalmology in Tampa to get his opinion about the hospital.

Hearing her audible apprehension raised mine again. I turned to Damion and asked, "Damion, are you urinating when you get up to use the bathroom?"

"Umm, no, not too much."

"D., do you know when the last time you peed was?

"I don't know," he answered distantly.

Not only did Grace sound worried but my conversations with Marnix were becoming more stressful. He was having mounting concerns. "I'm worried about the possibility of Crone's disease," he told me. What was Crone's disease? From his tone I was afraid to ask. "I'm not going to leave my room until this gets worked out," he went on. "I don't feel good about this doctor at all."

The Asian doctor returned in the early afternoon while I was immersed in one of the phone calls with my husband. I handed Marnix over to her again and listened to her side of the conversation. Her clipped but cheerful voice said, "Yes, that would show up in culture. Yes, yes, another CBC would be appropriate. No, he is doing very well and responding to IV fluids quite. . . . Yes, doctor. I will keep you posted."

At the end of this call I asked again about the blood. That question triggered a replay of the morning's reassurances. I persisted, to make sure she understood. "I'm not talking about a little blood," I said. "I mean a lot of blood."

This drew more platitudes. As she rattled on, I imagined how she would look at the tea party her smile suggested. Her black bun would be covered by a big bobbing hat with large pink cabbage roses on the brim.

"Please come look in the bathroom," I said. She followed, left the bathroom abruptly and did not speak to me.

LATE AFTERNOON

At about four o'clock Dr. Thaddeus Kiros entered Damion's room. He was in his fifties. "I was born in Greece and educated in Paris," he told me, in a reflective and calm voice. He was answering the Asian doctor's request for a consult. I liked the way he rubbed his chin and paused before he offered his thoughts. He did not shoot from the hip.

When Dr. Kiros had gotten the call on his beeper, he told me he was not going to take it, because it was late in his day and he wasn't on call any longer. But already being on the north side of town shopping for a car and not far from the hospital, he'd reconsidered. This will be quick, he had thought. His reconsideration was a pivotal moment. As evil can be revealed in inconsequential details, so can salvation. Dr. Kiros could in good conscience have turned the call over to someone else less qualified. Damion would have had to wait another day for the pediatric gastroenterologist. Precious time would have gone down the toilet, and time was bleeding Damion.

Dr. Kiros picked up a napkin from Damion's untouched tray and wrote three words in an orderly script. "This is not definitive," he said calmly. "We don't know how it could have happened or what the manifestations will be. I will talk further with you later"

I nodded. "Okay." To me, a strange syndrome—whatever it was—sounded better than a rare disease.

Taking my cue from his demeanor, I didn't ask questions, but as soon as he left I called Marnix and spelled out the words, "hemolytic uremic syndrome."

The only one who did well in all the developing commotion was Sebastian. Telephoning him, I caught him coming in from his afternoon tennis session and asked about his day. I listened absentmindedly about the sandwich he'd ordered at the outdoor cafe, about the lesson with Roland Jaeger, father of wunderkind Andrea, about how nice his coaches were, and no, he hadn't yet started on his school work. Now he was going out to swim with his new friends, but promised to get started with his books before dinner.

Calling the director of the camp, I explained my absence and asked if the coaches could continue looking after Sebastian until I could get back, hopefully this evening. In his friendly, laid-back Australian way he was very helpful, offering to see Sebastian through dinner and keep him in the dorm of full-time students until I returned.

With Sebastian's whereabouts settled, I turned my attention back to Damion and began to make more calls.

Jack Guggino was a friend of my family. He'd trained years ago under my father as a pediatric ophthalmology fellow. I'd met him during my rebellious, obnoxious teenaged stage. Once he'd taken me for a walk through our woods in Maine. His family had been staying at our summer house while my father lectured at near-by Colby College. Dr. Guggino was taking the course. Dr. Guggino was an all right guy, but I could tell he'd been recruited to talk some sense into an obstinate seventeen-year-old who didn't know where she was going.

I checked his number in the address book I always carried with me on trips and dialed. It was strange to be talking to Jack twenty years later in such a different, yet similar role. Clearly, I was lost again. He listened as I explained the helplessness of not knowing the hospital situation in a strange city, and of this tentative diagnosis of an illness we knew nothing about.

He offered his advice in a voice gathering force as he went on. "I'd move him to St. Joseph Children's Hospital. I'm on staff and I'll intercede to whomever you need if you move Damion. I'll call back later to check. Meanwhile, I definitely suggest you make plans to move him."

Hanging up, I felt as if his suggestion was actually a command.

Up to this point, the speed of events was manageable. I was the one who determined the pace, or at least I thought I did. I had decided when to travel, when to stop, and when to go for help. I had time to think about the problem. Even though it was complicated, the timing was doable. There was even time for me to use Damion's shower. While I was drying my hair, Dr. Kiros returned.

That's when my whole sense of time fractured.

"We need to move Damion immediately to a pediatric intensive care unit. I have arranged for transfer to St. Joseph Children's Hospital," he announced in a somber voice.

From this conversation on, I didn't think in terms of mornings, afternoons, or nights. Now, time was splintered into smaller pieces. That's what happens to time when things start crashing. An eternity can fill an hour when the presence of evil and danger smash into an afternoon.

To save him from repeating himself, I asked, "Could we get my husband on the phone?" He nodded and I dialed. Then I handed the telephone to him.

As Dr. Kiros related to Marnix the rapid drop in platelet levels over the last hours, I listened intently.

"Yes, it's quite dramatic and profound really. They've dropped from two hundred and eleven thousand to ninety-five thousand since he was admitted. BUN is thirty-two. Creatinine is rising. Obviously, renal failure is the immediate concern. White blood count is elevated. It's thirty-two point five. Dr. Heersink, he also has: fever, bloody diarrhea, and an elevated leukocyte count. Add to that the kind of ulceration and acute edema I see on his gastrograph along with the kidney dysfunction beginning, and we have severe problems. An ambulance should be here soon. Once he's moved, the other consults will make their assessments."

When I took the phone after Dr. Kiros left, Marnix's voice was taut enough to snap. "Mary, I can't find anything on this damn thing! But you know this is not good. Not good at all. . . ." His voice trailed off.

I had never seen my husband desperate in all our seventeen years together. On top of everything else, this in itself frightened me.

EVENING

I sat still, perfectly still, watching the slowly dripping intravenous fluid entering my son's vein.

In my mind I repeated, *Everything is good. Everything works. Everything can be fixed.*

Look, for instance, at this intravenous system. See how the Ringer's lactose fluid drips into clear thin tubing, then infuses into this perfect sleeping hand. The drops are uniform in size and precisely timed, hypnotic in their tempo. How? A little plastic wheel controls the rate. It's a simple and efficient design. Gravity and a little wheel, that's all it is.

What forces were being exerted on us? What wheel of fate was being turned for us now? "The rhythm of all this is getting out of control," I murmured. I tried to stop my whirling thoughts to focus once again on our past philosophy. *We can adjust the flow of events*, I thought. *We can slow it back down when we move Damion to St. Joseph's. Everything will be all right again.*

LATER IN THE EVENING

When Damion awoke, he held his right arm to his chest and rubbed his fingers together. It looked so strange to me. It was something I'd never seen him do. It was the motion of someone in deep turmoil.

"What is it, sweet boy? Are you thirsty?"

"Before we leave," he said, "I'm going upstairs."

His voice was conspiratorial, almost panting. His eyes darted excitedly.

"What do you mean, angel? There's nothing upstairs but more patient rooms. We have to stay in here and wait to be moved to the other hospital like Dr. Kiros told us."

He's waking from a febrile dream, that's it, I told myself, willing myself to be calm.

"Okay," he whispered.

I picked up the telephone. I planned to ask the camp director to change Sebastian from day student to full-time status until all this settled down. He had offered to help with whatever we needed, and there wouldn't be a problem.

"It'll only take a minute, Mom," Damion said suddenly.

"Damion, what are you talking about?"

"I'll be back in just a minute. I've been up there and I know where to buy it."

His fingers continued rubbing and trembling excitedly. I could only watch and wonder what he would say next. This was unbelievable.

"I'm going up to get this CD for my class. They'll really like it."

It took me a long time to move. *Maybe if I freeze in this position, I can erase this. If I don't respond, this tape will rewind and it won't ever have happened.*

"Mom, you'll really like it, too. Do you like this song right now?"

"Damion." My voice sounded normal to me. It belied the panic I felt. "I'll be right back."

As I backed from the room, I murmured to myself, "I am not going to run. I will simply walk past these ten rooms to the nurses' station. I will tell the nurses. I have been quiet and undemanding since we got here. I'm not going to panic or become demanding like the Mrs. Doctor they're waiting for me to be."

At the nursing station, they watched me as I spoke. "Damion's hallucinating."

They responded that they'd notify our pediatrician and Dr. Kiros about Damion's agitation and confusion. They did not return to the room with me.

Once back there, I looked more critically at Damion. His skin seemed somehow changed. Parched was too strong a word. Leathery was, too. There was a sort of diabolical sheen to his skin, like it had been thinned and rubbed with a cloth. What I noticed was too subtle to describe. You probably wouldn't detect it if he were not your child or if he were not acting strangely.

Quietly, I picked up the phone and dialed my husband's number once again. I whispered to Marnix what had happened.

"Get him out of there, Mary!" Marnix yelled.

I had to hold the phone away from my ear.

"Get him out of there, damn it! Why are you still there?" Marnix never cursed. He never yelled, either. "Kiros wrote his orders an hour and a half ago! I just talked to the doctors at St. Joseph's and they are lined up and waiting for him. Ask again about the ambulance. Ask them again, and please get him the hell *out* of there!"

Quickly, I walked down the darkening hall to the nurses' station where a gum-cracking desk nurse said, "Ma'am, all we can do is call the ambulance. We did that when Dr. Kiros ordered the transfer. We do not have many of our patients *leaving* in an ambulance. By the way, you need to get his records," the gum-chewing nurse added.

How could this woman chew gum when this was so important?

"Did you call Dr. Kiros a few minutes ago about my son's confusion?"

"We surely did," she said in a singsong voice.

"All right then. Where are his records?"

"You're going to need his x-rays, too."

"Yes, good. Right. I want everything. May I have them, please?"

"I'm sorry. We're understaffed right now."

Two nurses in a back corner of the station pivoted on their chairs to watch this. "You'll have to gather them up yourself. Radiology is in the basement. Medical records are on the first floor."

Bovine, that's what she was. I exhaled into myself. Her big vacant eyes were totally unconcerned. I whirled away and left her to chew her cud. I was certain I would never forget her or this hospital that wouldn't help us.

Racing back twenty minutes later with the manila envelope of film and all the charts I'd collected, I returned to Damion's room which was now completely dark. The phone was ringing, and Damion made no attempt to answer it. I can't remember who the caller was. From this point on, it rang a lot. There were calls from Marnix every few minutes, from Dr. Kiros, from Dr. Guggino who offered to meet me at St. Joseph's, calls from my sister Grace, from Dr. Forston in Dothan, and the doctors waiting at St. Joseph's. All of the calls had to do with me getting the show on the road. But I could do nothing except continue to ask at the nursing station for them to check on the ambulance.

Damion no longer slept. He shifted around the bed anxiously, rubbed his fingers, and tried to think straight. It was pitiful to watch how hard he tried. He asked a lot of questions about what time it was. He talked about how, if we were home, he'd have school today. Occasionally, his hands would relax and he would ask something completely out of context or improbable.

"When we watch Sebastian's tennis tomorrow, can I ride his bike?"

I tried to be comforting and calming. I did not try to correct his errors. I simply agreed with his statements and tried to keep the conversation pleasant and easy for him.

More calls came. Lots of calls. Everyone was angry now, most of all, Dr. Kiros and Dr. Plasencia who was waiting for us at St. Joseph's.

"Mary, how can you still be there? Let me speak with one of them myself," Marnix demanded.

I made another hike to the nursing station, where the clock read quarter after ten. Bringing one of the nurses back with me, I put her on the phone with Marnix. After no explanation about the five-hour delay, she handed the phone back to me.

"You have to get going."

"I will try, Marnix," I defended, not really thinking about his frustration. "But I cannot make the ambulance come." I watched Damion's urgent expression. He was desperate to interrupt. "Marnix, hold on just a second. What is it, D.?"

The nurse and I waited for what looked like an important announcement.

"It came."

Silence.

"What came, Damion?"

"The ambulance. It came in when you were out of the room. It landed on the sink."

"Oh, Marnix," I said, shocked. "You have no idea what's happening." I didn't want to say the word hallucinating with Damion lying there.

The nurse didn't try to hide her amusement. Her laughter stung Damion.

I had to leave so he wouldn't see me. What was going on? What was happening to Damion? What had infected my happy, normal boy of only a few days ago?

NIGHT

Now the Asian pediatrician was back. Her moonshaped, endlessly pleasant face looked worried now. She didn't talk much. She sat with me. Every once in a while, Damion woke and spoke of sights no one could see. A nurse came in and told me a helicopter was on the way to move Damion to downtown Tampa. When another half hour went by, I called the dispatcher myself. "What is wrong? I've waited six hours. My son is hallucinating. The pediatric intensive care unit at St. Joseph's has been waiting all this time. Why don't you come?" I couldn't help crying on the phone.

"Look, lady, all's we know is what the nurses tell us. A kid with diarrhea. We've had a couple of bad road accidents tonight and we have to assign vehicles in order of priority. A transfer with gastroenteritis comes after a crash on I-75."

The Asian doctor was becoming incensed with the nurses at last. She advised me to sign Damion out. "They've dragged their feet long enough," she said. "We'll get him into my car and move him ourselves, for gracious sakes!"

My watch read midnight. Just as we were planning how to transfer Damion ourselves, the sounds of wheels and metal shaking rolled down the hall. I saw in the doorway an ambulance gurney, low and compact. Two uniformed men steered it into the room, and with a simultaneous tug, the legs scissored up, and the gurney snapped to the height of the hospital bed. In one smooth arc of motion, Damion was lifted, covered up, and strapped onto this platform. There was the slightest pause at the end of this movement as they decided which paramedic would carry the IV bag. As efficiently as they'd entered, they began adroitly steering the gurney into the corridor.

Another pause.

"Oh, ma'am." One paramedic hesitated at the door as something caught his eye. "He might want those." He pointed to the back of the room.

There in the far corner were Damion's big, black basketball shoes. I grabbed them up. The Asian doctor excused herself as we followed the paramedics toward the nursing station. "I'll check up on you once you get settled into St. Joseph's." She paused. "Mrs. Heersink, I'm sorry it's been a trying evening."

"It's not your fault about the transfer," I told her. "Thank you for offering to help move him yourself. I don't know how you can work in this place."

She made no reply. As we maneuvered Damion into the elevator, the nursing staff sat staring at us from behind their station desk. No one jumped up to hold open the doors as they banged open and closed against the gurney. No extra hands appeared as we struggle with IV lines, the elevator buttons, and our belongings. No wish of good luck. Not a single kind gesture.

The shift had changed at 11:00. This was a new herd of noncommittal, vacant faces framed by the gaping elevator doors.

Three years later, the hospital would become the subject of national scrutiny and even jokes on late night television. One unfortunate patient had the wrong leg amputated there which sparked perennial debate on accreditation and medical incompetence in certain hospital centers. The surgeon blamed the nursing staff. No one, it seemed, could imagine how such a mistake could happen. No one, except Marnix and me.

In a hospital, everything that goes in must come out, usually through the emergency room. So here we were, rushing through the same corridors we had waited in last night. We passed Dr. Marinelli who was back on the overnight shift again.

"We're on our way to St. Joseph's," I explained to him quickly.

"I know," he said.

I wondered what he had suspected last night when he saw the blood and the films of the inflamed colon. Dr. Marinelli looked through me with a leveling stare. "I'll listen out for how he does."

After talking to him, I had to run to catch up with the paramedics.

"Thank you, Dr. Marinelli," I said, skipping backwards. "Thank you." I raised my hand toward him.

He waited in the hall expressionless, watching the doors erase us from his world.

As I rushed through the closing doors, I wondered what happened in cases like this. Did E.R. doctors think about the outcomes for the patients they tend to? Did they ever yearn for more continuity with their cases? Or, did they become E.R. doctors for the very reason they don't want to deal with patients beyond the initial care?

The ambulance ride was surreal. We cruised along the main highway that cut through rundown neighborhoods. To the south, low makeshift houses seemed tacked together, probably as materials to build them could be scrounged. Spiky tropical vegetation almost swallowed up the worst of the shacks but I could still see dirty, stained jalousie windows curtained with sheets, rotting and peeling structures, and rusted pickup trucks parked haphazardly in front yards. People slept in all those houses as we floated past, an ambulance with no siren, our flashing lights making emergency patterns dance on the exit signs. The light beams had an almost circus like gaiety about them as they swept over the streets.

We sat up high, the driver and I. Making small talk, the driver tried to make me feel better as I sat silent and stunned, staring out at the midnight misery. He told me about his kids. I tried to listen as he talked on and on about his boys, but my son was in the back with a paramedic fighting for his life. It was hard to acknowledge any other reality.

Suddenly we exited I-75 and slid into city traffic. Cars continued to defer to us as we approached a bridge with no shoulder lane. Hillsborough River, the small, green sign said as we glided over the bridge. The black waters below seemed immune to our dancing lights. Then we wheeled into the hospital driveway and drove around and backed up at a fluorescent opening under the raw red words, Emergency Department.

The elevator delivered us to the eighth floor where everything was hushed. The paramedics told me to wait with Damion outside two wooden swinging doors under a sign for the Pediatric Intensive Care Unit. I began reading the laminated instruction on the door, "Please use phone to call P.I.C.U. desk before entering." The doors swung open. The ambulance crew reappeared followed by a doctor and a younger man wearing scrubs.

"Mrs. Heersink, I'm Daniel Plasencia. This is Chuck."

It seemed to me that we were beginning all over again.

"I'd like you to describe Damion's symptoms," Dr. Plasencia asked. "When did all this begin? What has happened in the last hours?" Question after question about the mental deterioration as I voiced my hesitant answers. Dr. Plasencia didn't watch me at all, and I was glad he didn't. He was touching Damion, pinching the skin on the back of my son's hand, kneeling down on one knee to look into his eyes, running his hands up and down Damion's neck.

"Umm, hmm." He hummed in a Latin sort of way in response to pauses in my explanation. I knew he was listening to me, but the feel and sight of Damion consumed him. He touched him with gentle inquisitive fingers, searching and feeling with dark eyes. He was reading my son. I wondered what he was thinking.

Deep within, I began to pray. *Be the light at the end of our tunnel*, I thought. *Be the angel to whom Damion is entrusted*.

"Excuse us now, Mrs. Heersink. We'll get Damion settled, and we'll be out in just a few minutes." With that, Damion, Dr. Plasencia, Chuck, and the paramedics disappeared into the unit.

I stood leaning against the wall. It didn't look like a hospital here. Everything was soft, muted. The carpet and wallpaper were mauve. A procession of wall sconces lined each hall, giving off a diffuse, almost ceremonial light. It was quiet. In some places on the floor big squares of blue or green carpet tiles were inlaid in a scattered pattern. "I bet kids could jump hopscotch from one square to another," I murmured to myself. "This is nice up here, nice but lonely." The echoes of my voice intensified the feeling.

The paramedics came clattering back out the swinging doors, pushing their wheeled stretcher. They paused for just a moment to get my signature on their metal clipboard.

"Is this all I have to sign?" I asked, surprised that there were no forms to fill out, no insurance card to present. It was so hushed here. I longed for a human voice. I wished the driver could linger a few minutes. Now I wanted to hear his tales about his children, but they were off to their next assignment.

"Hope everything works out, ma'am," the driver called out from the elevator before the doors whooshed shut.

I was perfectly alone. I was profoundly alone. I could not remember the last time before all this began that people, especially children, were not surrounding me. And I could not recall ever being in this eerie kind of solitariness with a sense of being so far away, so utterly and firmly disconnected from everything which came before.

Late night hospital corridors are some of the few places in the modern world where one is plunged into true solitude. It's the kind of aloneness that primitive peoples live in, the kind of aloneness that would swirl around and settle into your soul on some ancient mesa, or that would be your last feeling as you dozed under a dense and rain-blackened canopy of ferns in a far off rain forest.

Eventually, Dr. Plasencia and Chuck returned, wheeling Damion out on a larger more complicated bed. Dr. Plasencia halted. "You can go down with Damion and Chuck for the CAT scan," he said softly.

I remembered that a CAT scan stood for Computerized Axial Tomography.

This is the kind of sci-fi medicine that can save him, I half thought, half prayed again.

The blond, "preppy-looking" technician grimaced. He was probably not too happy with us to begin with. Surely he'd been put on notice early in the evening that a pediatric patient was on the way from another hospital and scheduled for a scan. Now, many hours later, we dragged in just when he thought his work was drawing to an end uneventfully.

Marnix had griped to me about this kind of delay in his own practice. I'd heard all kinds of fuming complaints about patients coming in hours later than promised because the family stopped at McDonald's and the mall on the way in. Or detoured to pick up relatives four towns away, as long as they had the car out. I wanted to tell this angry young man that the delay wasn't my fault, but I'm not even certain it was us with whom he was angry.

Chuck got Damion settled onto the platform that slid in and out of the big doughnut-shaped machine. The CAT scan equipment consumed an entire room; the controls were in an adjacent space partitioned off from the machine. The terse man pointed for me to stand behind him at the keyboard. I could see Damion through a window. Chuck had obviously noticed my anxiety and asked this permission for me.

"Hold still now," the technician yelled through the partition.

The sliding platform obeyed rapidly typed commands. A bright beam projected inside the doughnut to reveal slices of Damion's skull. The cross sections of brain spread out in perfect precision across the screen. I couldn't believe that I was looking into my child's head!

Now some images were blurring as the beam scanned deeper sections of Damion's skull. "You've got to stop moving! Hold still now," the technician called to Damion.

"I'm just eating the last piece of my candy bar," Damion answered sheepishly as he hallucinated again.

Chuck went into the room to help. I heard him speaking calmly with Damion. "Hey, Buddy, stop chewing for just a minute so we can finish up these pictures. That's it. Let's see if you can stay very still. Just let it melt in your mouth slowly. Great, Damion, you're doing great."

Eventually, the technician seemed satisfied with the sharp films he was able to produce. He reviewed them, scrolling them across the screen quickly, his fingers flying across the keyboard. He was master of this incredible technology. His command printed the scans on glossy films that Chuck collected into Damion's file, and we were out of there.

"Thank you for letting me watch. I really wanted to see this. . . ." My words trailed off.

"Good night," the technician answered, his first and last words to me.

Dr. Plasencia asked Chuck to settle me in for some sleep. St. Joseph's had a couple of parent rooms adjacent to the pediatric intensive care unit. "We'll look after him and call if he needs you," Dr. Plasencia said reassuringly. "You look like you need some rest. How long has it been since you've slept?"

He'd caught me leaning on Damion's bed as we paused outside the P.I.C.U. doors. Chuck directed me to a room with its own telephone and bathroom. "These fold down and make beds. You can get sheets and towels from the linen cart in the hall. Here are some pillows in these drawers. You should be able to get some sleep in here. Good night now, Mrs. Heersink. We'll take care of him."

The clock mounted over the phone read two-thirty. It was the last thing I saw before I flipped off the light switch and fell into sleep.

In the darkness, I felt someone trying to wake me. My eyes caught the luminous green hands of the clock positioned at twenty to four. Dr. Plasencia was kneeling beside my bed. Chuck stood in the doorway shining a flashlight that sent yellow light into the dark. "Mrs. Heersink, we just want to let you know that Damion is sleeping. He has settled down. The CAT scans indicate no structural abnormality or intracranial catastrophe that can explain his mental deterioration. We are continuing to do blood and culturing work. We should have something more in the morning."

Then they departed. The room was dark again. I pulled the blanket over my head to make it blacker still.

6

Gathering

A team was being assembled. In our glassed-in corner of the pediatric intensive care unit, Damion and I were alone. I sat close to his bed, feeling guilty for having overslept until six-thirty that morning. He was sound asleep.

Damion, I thought as I watched him, *what's happened to you since last night? I hope you haven't needed me in this new nebulous space. Damion, no more than twenty feet away I see Dr. Plasencia behind the elevated desk area. Does he ever go home? He is pointing to your illuminated CAT scans. It's impossible that those black and white scans making a checkerboard of the wall are slices of your head! What has happened to the healthy boy you were only days ago? How can it be that you are the subject of this intense meeting?*

I know Dr. Plasencia is telling these men about you. There's nothing I want to do more than to hear what he is saying. But I don't want to put more pressure on him, so I'll keep my back toward the discussion, and face you, darling boy. I cannot help straining to catch the occasional word through the sliding glass door. They are talking about your lab work, talking on and on.

You can dream in this bright morning light. You don't have to agonize about all these numbers and all these men and all those scans on that illuminated wall. I'll do that for you, sleeping boy.

There were more voices now. I turned to catch a quick glimpse of the speakers. The group grew until it included six or seven people. They talked on and on. Then, over time, the conversation distilled down to two voices that seemed locked in debate. These two discussed something, their voices somber. Oh God, they talked such a long time. They used that acronym again, BUN. I heard "peritoneal" and "recommend." The flow of this exchange indicated a decision being made between a direct, athletic voice and a regal yet Americanized Middle Eastern accent.

Now Dr. Plasencia sounded like he was collecting the voices into one consensus. I heard him conclude, "Tell the mother."

He summoned me to the assembly and introduced me to the circle of doctors. All I could think was, *I'm never going to remember who's who.*

Dr. Plasencia handed me over to a solid, muscular man who had the direct tone in the debate moments before.

"This is Dr. Havis, pediatric nephrologist," he said.

Dr. Havis's personality was as direct as his voice. As he spoke matter-of-factly about the seriousness of Damion's condition, I thought, *I don't think this man is going to be my friend. It was not that he was unkind or cold, but I felt he was steeling himself towards me.* Then my heart constricted, as I thought, *There must be bad news coming. What was wrong with Damion?*

Dr. Havis cleared his throat. "We think this is H.U.S." His voice droned on and on, saying frightening words I didn't understand. "BUN should be in the 10-26 range. At Lennox Hospital it had risen to 32. This morning's latest lab work shows it is 54. His creatinine number is rising too. These numbers reflect that the kidneys are not functioning sufficiently to cleanse the blood of toxins. This probably explains Damion's confusion and disorientation. Meanwhile, urine output is decreasing. Dialysis is necessary."

I wanted to run away but stood riveted to the spot listening to words I wished I could shut out.

"Blood cells are being destroyed." He turned to me. "You need to prepare for the roller coaster ride of your life. One challenge after another may present itself. You make it through one descent and two others are on the horizon. This can go on for a long time."

I nodded. "But . . ."

Immersed in his explanation, he took no notice of my interjection. "This is a disease without a road map. Possible complications, aside from renal involvement, might occur in the digestive system, the pancreas, heart, lungs, and brain."

I tried to remain calm until Dr. Havis wound down his monologue with, "Mortality rates are something like. . . ."

This man was definitely not going to be my friend. Here he was making me cry in front of all these quiet, watchful doctors. I asked only one question. "What can you do to stop the blood cells from being destroyed?"

I felt my head swirling as he stated, "Nothing really. We had some discussion about plasma exchange therapy, but that has its risks and it is inconclusive whether it is beneficial. At this point the objective is to support with careful fluid management and dialysis."

Sensing that this concluded the purpose of having me join the group and aware that my hands were not doing an adequate job catching the tears falling down from my eyes, I said in a hoarse voice, "Please excuse me."

Out the double doors I spun, around one quick corner and into the first door on the left. Here I sat down on the foldout bed, crying.

Finally, fingers trembling, I dialed Marnix's number. The phone rang only half a ring before he picked it up. "Marnix, I know you have the exam today. I'm sorry." This was his child too. A tear fell onto the blanket as much for Marnix as for this boy we made.

"Please come now, Marnix. It's really bad. They think it's something called H.U.S. They're even telling me about mortality rates."

"I know."

He didn't say anything else. Just a long wet silence before he whispered, "I'll get the first morning flight to Tampa."

Terror. It was here now for the first time in our lives. It became our dread and loyal companion.

Terror was a hard crystalline lens through which everything passed. All decisions were magnified by it and loomed ominous and huge before us. Terror was a lens that condensed all our diffuse attentions into one precise focus: our boy's survival. All our energies were gathered and intensified by it into one burning beam. Nothing could distract us from this hot, white laser. Our other children, work, relatives, home, friends, obligations, sleep and hunger were all blurred into peripheral unimportance by our terror. Only the brilliant burning need of Damion mattered.

Terror was a powerful lens that refracted all the confusing new information and our scattered rays of emotion into one pure white will. It focused the absolute will that we needed for the ensuing battle.

It was a frightening, but useful ally.

Marnix and I admitted our panic to each other as we clung together verbally sharing our common misery on the telephone early the next morning. He told me he had been accommodating this great fear since yesterday evening when he'd looked up H.U.S. in his pediatric pathology texts and searched the medical school library for more material. The fear gathered force from my worsening reports of Damion's hallucinations and our delay in getting Damion transferred. Trapped in Birmingham, he'd felt the fear gnaw at him all night.

Marnix had memorized the flight number and the plane's departure time in the middle of the night.

My own part was easier than his, for I had at least been able to be with Damion to seek help for him at St. Joseph's whereas Marnix had to endure being far away and disconnected except by telephone. Yesterday had been so stressful and frightening. The frustration of Lennox Hospital was the worst part. Here at St. Joseph's all the people approached Damion with urgency and competence. I knew they would do their best to take care of him.

Most of all, I had it easier up to this point because of my ignorance. I had the bliss of not really knowing the deep recesses of medicine. I held the reassuring illusion that most people in the modern world harbor: medicine is almost limitless in its ability to diagnose and heal. "These are the days of miracles and wonders," as Paul Simon sang. Genetic interventions, magnetic resonance imaging, fetal surgery, and lasers made one feel that medicine could perform nearly any feat it put its mind to. Maybe it would not find the solution to AIDS by next year, but sympathetic as I was to that plight, it was never going to be my personal problem. At least so I believed.

If something was wrong, it could be fixed. This false faith was encouraged by my father's and my husband's work, and my perceptions of it. People didn't die at the hands of ophthalmologists.

Middle-of-the-night disasters didn't drag them out of bed. Marnix's cataract removals and my father's pediatric eye muscle repairs were scheduled surgeries, super-technical and successful. Afterwards, the operating floor did not need to be scrubbed of blood. Horrible news didn't need to be carried to family members. Nearly everyone could leave my father's or husband's care fixed and contented. Vision was restored. Filmy lenses were removed. Seniors could read and sew again. Eyes were straightened. Parents were happy. Everything worked out.

This overconfident creed of medicine as the great solution was an excruciating thing to surrender. Nevertheless, Dr. Havis's words, "mortality rates" began chipping away at my foolish faith. Still I tried tenaciously to hold into it.

Everything was good. Everything could be fixed. Everything worked.

These pillars of my faith were shaking precariously as I waited for Marnix to arrive in Tampa and get to the hospital. I waited to find out about the mysterious syndrome that might kill our son.

7

Intensive Care

PICKING UP THE PHONE outside the pediatric intensive care unit as the sign requested, I spoke: "Hello, this is Damion's mom. Is it all right if I come back in now?"

"Yes, that will be fine."

Entering the unit, I saw the woman who had just granted me permission. She was a tall woman with a blond beehive hairdo, undwarfed by the massive desk. She reigned over a bank of five or six monitors that looked like clones of Damion's personal computer back home. She was surrounded by several telephones and imposing communications equipment on the elevated desk. All of this was very impressive, very imposing, as were the four glass rooms that radiated out from this enormous enthroned woman.

"You need to wash your hands," her deep voice resonated.

"Oh, yes, ma'am," I said appropriately intimidated.

I walked inside Damion's cubicle and used his sink. I tapped the button on the wall-mounted dispenser of Hibiclens antibacterial soap, which dripped out. I washed my hands and dried off with paper towels mounted on the wall. I wondered why she was so concerned about my hand washing. I had no idea how much we'd use the sink in the time to come.

Damion was quiet but alert. His skin seemed stretched, yet, other than his bulging belly, he didn't appear to be bloated. He had a second IV now on his other hand.

A tube had been threaded into his nose, down the back of his throat, and through his esophagus into his stomach. Terri, his pert, bouncy nurse, walked up. "It's a naso-gastric tube, or NG tube," she said as if that were self-explanatory. The clear tube was taped in place where it entered his left nostril. Greenish brown liquid was slowly winding its way from his stomach to an apparatus on the wall behind him. It made a swishing vacuuming sound as it occasionally sputtered drops of green liquid into a clear plastic dispenser.

"Bile," I said tentatively.

"Yes, bile," Terri answered. "He hasn't had anything to eat for what did you say, three and a half days now? So that's all bile. He'd be nauseated and very uncomfortable without this and the Zantac we're giving him." She turned toward the bed and said, "It wasn't fun putting it into place, but now that it's there, your belly feels better, doesn't it, honey?"

Damion nodded. I liked the way she involved him in what was happening to him, rather than just intruding on his body. Thank God he was not a toddler who could never understand.

Terri now placed on his index finger an alligator-jawed clamp which had one bulb that lighted up red. Then she plugged the wire to the clamp and plugged the other end into the television monitor over Damion's head.

"E.T.," she teased him. "That's your E.T. finger, glowing just like in the movie."

She moved around constantly to adjust the finger light, punching buttons on the screen that had now come alive to show a fluctuating white numeral. At intervals she recorded the amount of urine collecting in a transparent vinyl bag that hung on the side of the bed.

But I couldn't help wanting to feel some part of him, to hold my boy, so I grasped a section of the tubing coming out from his sheets. I could feel the warmth of the fluid through the cool plastic.

Meanwhile, Terri was peeling paper backings from round, skin-toned patches that had metal nipples in their centers. She continued explaining everything to us, giving the impression that all of this was no big deal. "Oh, we're just going to stick on these funny patches that will show you how fast your heart is beating and what your blood pressure is."

She untangled a group of thin tan cords and clamped the electrodes one at a time to Damion's patches. Then she plugged the free ends into the monitor overhead.

"Damion, you are now online. Your E.T. light tells how much oxygen is in your blood. Yep, that's right. Oxygen is the number ninety-six in the corner. How did you know O-two stands for oxygen? Dog, boy, you know a lot. We are definitely going to get along. I just love smart patients.

"And the electrodes tell the computer what your heart rate is. It's the red number that's blinking from one-seventeen to one-thirty. Now, see the blue numbers? They're your blood pressure. That's right, one-forty over ninety. And that last number tells us how many breaths a minute you are taking, twelve to fifteen."

Terri kept up this one-sided conversation, which helped calm me. When she talked about her own eleven-year-old boy named Robbie, she rubbed Damion's leg as if it were her son's. She combed his hair so that, she said, "You can keep on looking handsome this morning."

She brought him Styrofoam cups of ice chips when he began complaining about thirst. Finally he begged to drink, thank God. That must be a good sign, I thought. I looked at her, hoping she'd say something comforting but she only cautioned him, "Not so fast, sweetie. You can only wet your lips with it."

At mid morning, Dr. Plasencia came in and sat on the edge of the bed. He had many questions, but first, he examined Damion's abdomen. It was distended. Sometimes when the children were toddlers, I'd notice after a big dinner that their bellies would bloat. But never this much. You could never eat enough food to make your abdomen as full and tight as Damion's. It looked like a drum and had to hurt, I thought. Dr. Plasencia rubbed his hands together to warm them, then began to palpate firmly just below Damion's rib cage. "How does this feel, Damion? Any pain there?"

"Not really."

"And down here, around your belly button?"

Damion sucked in his breath and raised his hands off the bed to guard his belly. The doctor's hands were gentle but firm on the lower quadrants of his abdomen.

"No, no, no!" His hands grabbed Dr. Plasencia's wrists. "Please don't touch me there. That hurts too much!"

Dr. Plasencia swung his legs toward my chair.

"I want to ask you a few questions. Have you traveled to a

foreign country recently?"

"We go to Holland in the summer," I said slowly. That didn't satisfy him.

"I'm looking for a specific kind of country. Has Damion visited South America or an undeveloped nation in the last few months?"

All sorts of exotic bacteria, tropical viruses and parasites sprang to mind, and dangers that weren't part of my world whirled through my thoughts.

"No, sir." My mind started to slide. I wondered to myself if yesterday's hospital would qualify as underdeveloped.

Plasencia's voice broke into my thoughts. "Is he around livestock or farm animals?"

"We have new puppies." Again that didn't make an impression on him.

"Or has anyone else in your family had any gastrointestinal illness?"

"No." I shook my head. I tried to think back and came up with nothing.

"Are there any genetic blood disorders in the family? Any clotting diseases? Cystic fibrosis?"

"No," I said. "Nothing on either side."

"Have there been any changes in Damion's environment or activities in the last few weeks?"

I felt like I was being interrogated and failing to satisfy the interrogator. "I don't think so. I can't think of anything different."

"Does he drink unpasteurized milk?"

"Never."

"Do you have a septic tank, or are you on a city sewage system?"

"City."

"Has Damion had pneumonia or other respiratory problems?"

"No. He's never been sick before. He's been a very robust child."

Though Dr. Plasencia came up empty-handed, I got the impression that he thought we'd been exposed to something amazing like the plague in the previous week. Family history, our habits, none of my answers helped him. Finally, he got up from the edge of Damion's bed and walked over to the tall woman's desk. I watched him lean over charts, give instructions on the phone, check papers for nurses, and confer with doctors who came into the unit to be updated on the other children's progress. My eyes didn't leave him as he wrote, called people, ordered x-rays and tests and read the constant lab reports that were handed to him by the large stationary woman. He was successfully juggling the care for all of these sick children. Terri told me there were four intensive care patients on our side and six or seven on the other side of the hall. Dr. Plasencia orchestrated the care for them all.

"Why's the pediatric intensive care unit split?" I asked Terri, who I sensed was glad to change the topic, glad I hadn't voiced the overwhelming but unasked question: what is going to happen to my child?

Terri answered the question I did voice.

"Originally, it was intended for that side of the unit to be intensive care and this side to be progressive care. That turned out not to be practical, so now we have essentially two sides of intensive care. When it's not busy, we shut one down."

I nodded but didn't pay much attention to her words. I couldn't think about anything except Damion. I had to try to understand all that was happening. "Terri, may I ask you some things? This seems like a good time now that he's dozed off, and you don't look as busy as you were earlier with him."

"Sure."

"I really don't understand the kidney and fluid situation. For one thing, why does he have two IV's now?"

"One IV gives him fluids only. The other gives him fluids and is reserved to give him meds. Danny says he's quite dehydrated." From conversations I had overheard I knew that Danny was Dr. Plasencia.

"But he's been on IV fluids since he went to University Community Hospital. Shouldn't that have helped him avoid dehydration?"

"What Damion received wasn't enough to make up for his deficit from the diarrhea and lack of fluid intake. See how dry his skin is? And his eyes are sunken? When Danny inserted the NG tube, there were no tears when he cried. We're trying our best to rehydrate him, but it's tricky because of his kidney situation."

"I learned it when I took physiology
forgotten that now. What's the BUN acronyi.

"Blood urea nitrogen. Its level shows
clearing the body's waste products from the
range is from ten to twenty-six. Yesterday it wa.

"Thirty-two when Dr. Kiros reported it to   ..ie
afternoon."

"And Dr. Havis told you that on admit it had risen to fifty.
That's one reason we're doing blood work so often, to follow BUN
and creatinine, another renal indicator. One of the most important
things with renal failure is fluid management. Dr. Havis and Danny
are watching that very carefully, ordering a renal sonogram to see
what kind of damage the kidneys show, and lining up dialysis that
will take over the work his kidneys aren't able to do now. And
because the kidneys have caused his blood pressure to elevate,
they're giving him Procardia to keep that from rising dangerously."

"Sounds like a delicate balancing act."

"That's about it," she nodded.

"Terri." I paused and expressed another fear. "Why is the
urine in that bag so dark?"

She looked up and said somberly, "The kidneys aren't
putting out much volume. Damion's getting Lasix in his IV line to
encourage urine output. We don't want the kidneys to shut down
and not put out anything. We need to keep everything open."

One of the IV bags began to beep softly indicating it was
empty. Terri got up to replace it. She worked deftly and calmly as
though she could hold everything in balance for Damion.

I knew it would take more, but I said, "Thanks, Terri. I know
you're busy, but this helps me a lot to understand a little of what's
going on inside him."

"You hang in there. Now what time did you say your husband's plane will arrive?"

"In a couple of hours. Ten o'clock or so."

I asked, "Terri, how important is it that my husband be here
this morning as opposed to this afternoon?" I was feeling momentarily guilty about calling Marnix and forcing him to cancel out of
his exam. Now I felt lulled by the calm nature of Damion's morning
in Terri's care.

She stared at me as if I still didn't understand. "He needs to
here," she said ominously.

Soon Damion woke needing to use a bedpan. Terri helped
him onto it, edging it under his sheet. A surge of diarrhea began.
Dr. Plasencia appeared and said to Terri, "Weigh the bedpans."
Confirming large amounts of clotting blood, he sent samples to the
lab for culture.

Soon the bloody mess began pouring out of Damion with
such intensity that it seemed his intestines had ruptured. There was
no deference to teenaged modesty by morning's end. Each time the
explosion came, Terri remade the bed while I washed Damion.
Sheets and towels became a mound in the corner. Finally, someone
discreetly parked a laundry hamper outside our glass door. The
water ran bright red as I wrung out washcloth after washcloth in the
sink. Each time there was more hemorrhage than diarrhea. The
mess was shocking in its volume and bloodiness.

A repulsive foreign odor mixed with the blood smell. It was
not a fecal one. It was the odor of something vile and invasive—the
revolting smell of evil. Whatever was invading Damion I smelled in
the bloody sludge. Soon I detected this odor on his skin and on his
breath, even his hair. To me it was heinous. The smell was alien. It
was pervasive. Something horrible was strengthening in its host, my
boy's body.

This was also the beginning of his furious thirst. Damion
had nothing to eat or drink since Friday evening other than a few
reluctant sips of fluids. Now, more than three days later, his lips
were crusted, his throat parched. The constant diarrhea, the intermittent fever, and the turmoil of an unstable renal picture left him
very weak and depleted. This dehydration unbridled a wild physio-
logical need. That dehydration was a savage force breaking through
with a vengeance.

By midmorning it consumed him. He begged and begged for
relief. Terri brought out little pink glycerin sponges on lollipop
sticks that we moistened for him. He could have a damp rag in his
mouth, but we had to stop the ice chips.

Dr. Plasencia explained apologetically, "He can't have any
more ice because of the general anaesthesia with his surgery this
afternoon."

Upon these instructions, Terri quietly wrote big on a large piece of paper, "NPO" and taped it under his monitor.

As his thirst grew, so did Damion's disorientation. Dr. Gunderman, a large and jovial man, was called in. He was introduced to me as a pediatric neurologist. Gunderman checked Damion's pupils, reflexes and general neurological responses. I was glad to see Damion laugh a little in response to seeing the doctor's bag, which was filled with as many tattered stuffed animals as it was with medical paraphernalia.

Towering at the foot of Damion's bed, he asked, "You see this monkey? He has been all over the hospital. Every time Danny's son, who's the same age as you, is up on the floor, he steals my monkey and hides it somewhere in the building. Once it ended up in the laundry. Another time, the janitors found it in the service elevator. Everyone knows it belongs to me and I get it back. Just look how beaten up this thing is."

Before leaving the unit, Dr. Gunderman took me aside. "Damion's confusion," he reassured me, "is likely due to his kidney dysfunction and the toxins that consequently are backing up in his bloodstream."

When we were alone again, Damion kept asking me questions about what time it was. He was trying to orient himself to combat the confusion. "It's Tuesday morning," he kept repeating. Sometimes the big clock on our wall steadied him in this desperate effort to stay grounded, although because it looked like the clock in his classroom, sometimes it only confused him more.

"And it's March 3, because March 1 was Sunday, and March 2 was Monday, and it's not Monday anymore. So it's eleven o'clock and it's Tuesday, Mom. Right?"

"You're right, Damion. Absolutely."

"And on Tuesday, we don't have P.E. after lunch."

And so we managed the morning. Blood flowed down the sink. I distracted him from his thirst and he talked valiantly about how it was Tuesday.

Suddenly I saw a familiar tall dark suit through the tilted blinds on our sliding door. Marnix at last! I jumped up to hug him. "Oh, your papa is here!" I cried to Damion. Thank God, I murmured. Dr. Plasencia came to our cubicle and introduced himself to Marnix. Marnix spoke to Dr. Plasencia just long enough to be polite and then rushed to Damion's side. Dr. Plasencia returned to the desk, I suppose to give us a few minutes as a family.

"Animal," Marnix smiled before he hugged Damion.

I loved it when Marnix nicknamed Damion "Animal." Sometimes during basketball games, Marnix would shout out, "Yes! Animal! Way to rebound!" It was so embarrassing to Damion, but endearing to me.

"How are you doing, sweet boy?"

"Aren't you going to take your test this morning, Papa? It's March 3. It's Tuesday."

"I know, baby. I wanted to come see you instead."

I watched my husband and son and silently prayed, *Thank you, God, for giving Damion the most wonderful father in the world and for giving me the best husband, and for getting him here to lean over Damion's bed to comfort him.* Marnix was able to do certain things. He brought out certain things in our children that I couldn't. I realized how much we needed him here.

Soon, Marnix was meeting all the doctors. He wrote down numbers and notes. He asked many questions about the values, the tests, the plan for Damion. He was included in their conferences. He was gracefully allowed in as a member of the team. Is it an asset to have a physician in the family? Obviously, Marnix's presence improved our information and involvement. Even care, perhaps. But this was indirect and never intentional. Was this unfair? Of course it was. But that morning I gratefully accepted the inequity and thanked God that Damion was on the right side of unfairness.

Meanwhile, another white-garbed figure tapped my shoulder. "Surgical consent forms? Yes, I'll sign them. My husband is busy with Dr. Havis and Dr. Plasencia."

I signed the paperwork. Then there were a portable chest x-ray and a renal ultrasound to be accomplished before surgery. As soon as the operating room and the surgeon were available later this afternoon, Damion would have a catheter implanted into his abdominal space under general anesthesia. The catheter would allow dialysis to begin.

I don't know precisely when it was that I started calling Dr. Plasencia Danny. It was hard not to. Terri and the other unit nurses referred to him by his first name all the time. By late afternoon, Damion was calling him Danny, and Dr. Plasencia did not object. It was inevitable that we would use his first name also, although he never invited us to. I don't think it was because Marnix was there nor that doctor-to-doctor rapport allowed it. I just think no one could be around the doctor for more than half a day and not feel comfortable and close enough to this elegant yet approachable man to, without thinking about it, call him Danny.

When Marnix wasn't talking to Danny, he sat with Damion and helped to keep him clean and calm. He tried to steer Damion's thoughts away from his thirst by telling him stories or asking questions about players on his soccer team. Sometimes Marnix left for a few minutes to make phone calls.

During one of these trips, I noticed Damion becoming more and more agitated. He started to cry, "Please get me something to drink. Give me a quarter and I'll get a Sprite," he said hoarsely. I tried to placate him but all my explanations and excuses only made him angrier and more insistent.

Finally I ran out to the bedroom the hospital had given me to get Marnix and said, "Marnix, can you come? He's crying and begging for a drink."

Marnix's finger raised in the signal "wait," so I went into the bathroom and splashed some cool water on my face. Through the open door I could see Marnix hunched over on my bed, snapping his pen nervously against his shoes over and over.

"Well, okay," he was saying on the phone. "Oh, ma'am. Ma'am? Perhaps I could leave a message for him. His associate? Yes, please, I'll talk to him."

I looked into the mirror at my unkempt reflection. Maybe I have time to brush my teeth, I thought distractedly.

Marnix was talking, trying to sound calm but not succeeding. "Yes, hello. This is Marnix Heersink. I'm an old friend of John's from medical school. My son has been diagnosed with hemolytic uremic syndrome. The secretary told me that John is out of the country. Will he be back any time soon? Two weeks? Yes, just in case, it's Heersink, H-E-E-R-S-I-N-K. Heersink. Listen, just off hand, what is John's approach on therapy? I understand. Aggressive. Jump on it. Got it. Well thanks. Thank you. If he calls in, I'd appreciate it. Goodbye."

I came out of the bathroom. "Marnix, what can we do? It's getting to be agony for Damion. Now he's begging for quarters to go buy a Sprite. Who was that?"

"Never mind, it didn't work out. I just have a lot to think about in terms of treatment for him. Come on, let's go back. Let's see what we can do to keep him settled till they take him down to surgery," he answered sadly.

After granting us permission to reenter, the imposing, granite-like woman decreed once again, "You have to wash your hands."

By now I knew her name was Alice.

"Yes, Alice, I know. We always do."

"No, not in there. *Here.*"

Alice rose majestically and marched over to us. At the door she showed us the sink we had bypassed in our haste. She demonstrated how to operate the faucet by stepping on the floor lever. Although Marnix had two of these very same sinks mounted in the passage between his two operating rooms back home, he nodded as though he'd never before seen such a clever apparatus. It was best to submit to Alice, I thought.

"Oh, sorry, I didn't see this sink," I murmured. And I hadn't, although I'd passed by it now at least ten times. Before Alice had politely allowed us to skip over the rules and use Damion's sink. But now that it looked as though we were settling in, she had to enforce protocol. Obviously, infection is a constant threat in an environment where children are so compromised. I looked over at the space where one baby slept under a plastic tent with a mass of air hoses over its crib.

"Thank you, Alice."

She smiled regally and strode back to her lookout station.

"I'm sorry," Terri was saying to Damion, and she really was. "We've got to do this, Damion darling. If you try not to pull on these, we'll keep them as loose as we can, honey."

She looked at us apologetically as we entered. "I hate tying

Damion's wrists to the bed," she said. It seemed that while we were out of the P.I.C.U. and Damion was left alone for just a few seconds, Terri had returned from grabbing more clean linens to find him standing up on his bed. He had disconnected the electrode wires and was trying to rip out his IV lines.

"I'm going down the hall to buy a soda from the drink machine I saw there," Damion had announced to Terri. Now he was in restraints.

"Oh, baby, please don't cry. I'm going to read you this magazine I brought you from the plane. Mom's wringing out a damp cloth for your mouth. Here are some pictures of futuristic cars I want to show you." Marnix tried to keep him distracted.

Every hour was twice as hard as the one before. It became one o'clock. Then two o'clock. They'd take him to surgery soon, I hoped. It became three o'clock. Damion insisted, "I have a cooler under this bed. It's filled with Sprites and Minute-Maids. Why can't I just drink them? They're mine! Why are you hiding them from me?" Agony swept through me. It became four o'clock.

"Please untie me!"

The glass door slid open and shut as Dr. Plasencia and the nurses came in and out to check on him. Alice often looked up from her work toward our cubicle. Janitors, other children's nurses, and parents glanced furtively into our space as they passed. Damion screamed, cried, begged, and pleaded. When we could convince him that we weren't conspiring to deny him a drink, that he couldn't drink because he was going to surgery soon, he had us make a list for him. He dictated the drinks he wanted, listed them in the order that he would drink them, made us write down the size container, made us write down how much ice to put in each one. We tried to read to him and distract him, but he'd cry and make us rewrite the list. He'd revise it. This time he wanted two Sprites first, then one glass of water.

"Christ Almighty, this is torture. Marnix, while Terri is out of the room give me that cup. Damion, suck on this one piece. Four o'clock will be here soon, then they'll take you downstairs. Daddy and I will come with you. Make this piece last, baby."

I knew this was wrong, but one piece of ice was not going to hurt him during the surgery. It's not like he was going to vomit up one melted ice chip and inhale it into his lungs, I thought. Marnix perhaps knew better, but he didn't try to stop me.

Damion was red and parched and rasp-voiced now, trapped in his hellacious thirst. The ice chip meant everything to him. He closed his eyes and relished it.

"Thank you, Mom. Thanks." One hot tear ran down his cheek.

Dr. Gunderman came in. "Try and keep him oriented," he said quietly. "Part of Damion's agitation is frustration with losing his grip on reality." Damion looked to us to help him keep his balance, to steady him. Dr. Plasencia took the same approach. Every time he came in to wait with us he'd speak to Damion in a kind, but commanding way. Damion responded well to this.

But for us as parents, this became more impossible as the torturous afternoon ground on. Damion's tenuous grip on reality was slipping away. His eyes filled with panic. Sometimes he believed he was on Matt Hall's playroom couch, playing Nintendo on what was in reality the monitor screen beeping above him.

Once Dr. Gunderman asked, "Who's this, Damion?" as he pointed to me.

Damion puzzled over this, determined not to be trapped by this question. Not embarrassed any longer, only angry at all of us, he blurted out, "Lee!" Lee was a boy that sat beside him in the sixth grade.

None of us could do anything but wait and try to comfort him. There was nothing anyone could give him to subdue the violent thirst. Marnix explained to me that a child in such flux, hours before going under general anesthesia, could not safely be sedated. By the time the orderlies came to get our son, we were white-knuckled from the wreckage of the last hours. A demon raged inside our boy's body, and we could only watch in awe of its violent nature.

Oh, Damion, please do well in surgery, please do well with the anesthesia. Please do well, our baby, we thought but never said as we kissed him at the O.R. doors. When the scrub nurse checked his hospital I.D. band against the operative chart, we thought but never said, Please don't be one of the children that doesn't wake up.

Aloud we said, "Mommy and Daddy love you so much. All these people will take very good care of you while you sleep."

Marnix and I found our way to an empty waiting area, where we tried to untangle our mutual fears. Here, we had the first quiet time alone to help each other with our knotted anguish. As much as we dreaded Damion being under anesthesia and having to go through the trauma of surgery now, we prayed this would keep him alive.

After a few minutes, we didn't talk anymore. Marnix spent the time writing notes and questions on his tablet, and rubbing his forehead. I struggled with one leaden question: How in hell's name could this be happening to our child? Time dragged by. Finally, it was over.

The recovery room nurses waited until Damion was extubated. Then, Dr. Swank came to talk to us. We had met Dr. Swank earlier in the afternoon when he spoke with us briefly about the surgery. It was all mysterious to me how the dialysis would actually occur through a catheter lodged in Damion's peritoneal cavity. With Marnix's understanding of the process, with Damion requiring total attention at that point, I prayed it would all somehow work out. I told myself, Here was this upright, obviously competent, pediatric surgeon who would be in control. The nurses and Dr. Plasencia assured us that Dr. Swank was a superb surgeon. Dr. Swank looked surprisingly like the photographs of my father in his forties. His manner was very much like my dad's, too. All of this added up to a sense of trust in this man and what he would do to help Damion.

"Everything went well. You can be with him now."

Dr. Swank was not a man of extra words. As Marnix asked him about the details, I gathered up Marnix's jacket and papers off the Naugahyde seats. I felt myself free-falling into gratitude. Damion had made it through the preliminary loop of his roller coaster ride! *Thank you, God, thank you for letting him continue to live.*

Marnix and I entered the large tiled recovery room. All the surfaces and equipment, even the nurses' scrubs were either blue, gun metal gray, or gleaming stainless steel. Damion was the only patient left this evening in the Recovery Room. There were four or five nurses trying to wrap things up at the end of their long day. But first, they needed to observe this one child until he was ready to go back to P.I.C.U. That would take about forty-five more minutes, which they spent putting things away, organizing the curtained spaces where empty gurneys were parked, changing linens, and checking over equipment.

As we approached Damion, the casual banter among the women suddenly stopped. One nurse, a stoic looking black woman, gazed at us. Her look froze me. Her doleful expression was one of lacerating sympathy. It was one of those injuring, incisive moments that told me this was truly bad . . . big trouble.

Damion's eyes were closed under a smear of Vaseline. He had rapid eye movements under the trembling lids as if he were in some netherworld. Bluish spots called petechia were developing where his skin was rubbed. His whole body shook every few seconds in a shiver. The tremors were a part of emerging from the anesthesia. Marnix lifted the sheet covering our son. Now, besides a tube up his nose, two IV lines, electrodes on his chest, a urinary catheter, and a subclavian line threaded into his right upper chest tacked down with stitches, in addition, Damion had a transparent tube sewn into his lower belly. His abdomen was so remarkably distended that the puffy incision looked like it would split.

Oh, D.D., now they're cutting you, I thought. The sight of his angry wound penetrated me.

"Precious, it's okay. You did just perfectly. Everything is fine, sweet boy. Daddy and Momma are going to stay with you. Do you want Papa to rub your head like this?"

A deeper shiver and a quickening of his heart rate on the monitor were his reply.

Dr. Plasencia and the nurses brought their sleeping patient back to P.I.C.U. In the ensuing hours, as we watched Damion sleep off the anesthesia, we fixated on the numerals on the monitors. They were to become the source of our relief or our agony.

He was undergoing the first phase of dialysis. A lot rested on its success. It had to remove the life threatening toxins and wastes accumulating in his blood.

Dialysate liquid was being infused into Damion's abdominal

cavity, or peritoneum. There it collected some of the dangerous waste and was flushed back out. As I watched, I saw that what went in clear came out blood-tinged a dramatic pink.

All of this had to be conducted with strict sterile technique. Terri wore a surgical mask and gloves and took great pains to make sure the portals on the bags and tubing remained untouched during connection. We had to don masks and stand back. Contamination would gain easy entry into Damion's abdominal cavity if there was any degree of carelessness. He could not afford infection.

Marnix turned towards me. "You should sleep a few hours while everything is calm and he is sleeping."

I started to protest but Marnix went on. "You have to get some rest. Now that Terri's leaving, I'll stay with him until after the next shift change."

Terri had worked a double nursing shift for us, since she knew the operation of the dialysis machine better than the other nurses. It had been a very long day for her, too. She looked as tired as I felt. As she cleaned up the paper and plastic from the last sterile pack, she agreed. "That's a good idea, guys. I'm going to stay long enough to be sure the next shift is very comfortable with the machine. I won't leave until then. Take turns getting some rest. Parents need sleep too, you know. Damion looks peaceful now after such a rough day, doesn't he?"

"All right," I said, "I'll get some sleep and then I'll relieve Marnix after midnight. We'll take turns sitting with Damion through the night."

I lay down. Sleep overpowered me immediately. A deceptive sleep that dissolved this new reality into a nightmare. In my dream, Damion was in trouble, we were in trouble, but the problem was reconstructed into a maze from which I searched for a way out. I relived the day, but abstractly, on my terms, aloof from the reality of the disease and Damion's danger.

Suddenly, Marnix's hand was on my shoulder, and I had to leave my search. Swimming back up to wakefulness was painful, not so much because I was tired and deeply asleep, but because of a reluctance to return to a more threatening reality from which there might be no exit.

The nightmare we were living.

"Mary, can you get up now? Damion is still peaceful. Stay with him. I don't know about this new nurse. Watch her. Wake me if the numbers change. Sorry, I just can't stay awake any longer."

His voice trailed off, exhaustion overtaking him. We spoke in the kind of shorthand close couples use in times of crisis. Without elaborating, both knowing what we weren't saying.

"Here are the ranges we talked about today. I made a list for you. Make sure Damion's numbers stay within these limits. If they don't, come and get me."

"Go to sleep, Marnix. Don't think about today. Tomorrow's got to be better. It certainly couldn't be worse, could it?"

"Oh my God," Marnix sighed, the pillow now over his head. "Call me, Mary. *Call* me if any numbers change." As I closed the door leaving the room, I hoped his dreams would be as deceptively hopeful as mine.

It was amazing that we could sleep, yet necessary. Never having been seriously sleep deprived in my life, I was learning it was possible to function for a day or two with hardly any rest. But after that I became useless. My mind turned to rubber. I found myself staring stupidly at people talking to me. I could not think clearly anymore. I couldn't even feel emotions after a certain amount of deprivation. From now on, I vowed, Marnix and I would sleep in shifts and allow each other to get a couple of hours respite here and there.

Sitting with Damion that night, everything was quiet in the unit. None of the monitors from the other children beeped. Damion slept. I tried in vain to read the same pages I had in the other hospital's emergency room. (*How long ago was that? It seemed eons ago and yet was only yesterday.*)

Time was a continuum with no clear definition of day or night, wakefulness or sleep. One of its strange effects was difficulty remembering the sequence of events. Tonight I resolved to gather up everything. Write it down. Basic trends in lab results, abbreviated notes on which doctor said what. This would help orient me, I felt. A day and a half later I abandoned the project. It proved too daunting. It was hard enough to live these events, much less take the time to record the salient points of every complication that arose.

The monitor beeped and buzzed reassuringly at low volume. There was only the occasional disturbance of a new IV bag being hung, or an adjustment of Damion's oximeter, the "E.T." light on his finger. How different this all was from this afternoon when we'd watched our son driven to madness by thirst and the poison in his blood.

Only the nurse who occasionally came into our cubicle worried me, as she had Marnix. As she pounded about performing her feats of caretaking, she did not inspire confidence. I say "feats" because she was so tremendously obese that moving across the room was a labor for her. She grunted and sighed and breathed so loudly while she banged around the dimmed space that I grew concerned for her health also.

However, concern for her soon developed into distress for Damion as I watched her fiddle with the dialysis machine. She poked the buttons with tentative fingers, gave a grunt of frustration, and left. When she returned, she had an operator's manual which she spread out on Damion's blanketed feet to study. When she finally figured out the programming, her next step was to replace the bags of dialysate. Spreading out a sterile paper on which to work, she put on surgical gloves and got me to mask up. All of this looked right. But I couldn't believe it when I saw her tug and grunt, trying to pull a clamp off one of the bags. Then she yanked it out with her teeth! *I couldn't believe she did that!* But I decided to keep quiet because her mouth was inches away from the exposed porthole. Then she began to detach the used dialysate bag, which was tinted pink with blood. I watched again in amazement as she yanked and yanked on its clamp. One tug was too forceful. The fluids spattered on Damion's face and the sheets. He slept through it, but I was horrified at the sight of him drenched with dialysate fluid, stained by his own toxins and blood.

"Don't you have to be really careful of contamination when you change the bags?" I finally said, through my clenched teeth.

A frown of concentration and a grunt were her only reply as she finished the task. Then came a major bed changing effort to clean up the spill. Because of all the tubes and lines we needed to untangle as we slid sheets under them, Damion stirred and moaned during this unnecessary disruption. For the remaining hours of the night, I thought of obscene adjectives to complete Marnix's description: "I don't know about this new nurse."

At 7:00 A.M. when Terri returned to duty, I confided in her what I'd seen. Terri passed it on to Dr. Plasencia and never again did that night nurse reappear on our side of the unit.

8

Platelets and Plasma

EARLY WEDNESDAY MORNING, March 4

When I returned to the unit, Damion appeared to me to be more stable than yesterday. His thirst didn't roar. He mostly slept. "And he's better oriented when awake," I said to Marnix, searching his face.

"The dialysis has begun to help his kidneys, yet his BUN over the last twenty-four hours has risen from fifty-four to seventy-eight." Marnix shook his head.

I shuddered. My initial optimism was fading. I knew peritoneal dialysis wasn't like turning on a light inside Damion. It wouldn't change the chemistry of what was happening inside him. Processes in the body were complex. They were interdependent. They took time to heal.

"Hematologically, he's in increasing danger." This was Marnix's immediate concern.

So began the day of platelets and plasma.

Normally, Damion would have a platelet count of 130,000 to 400,000. At the other hospital they'd declined from 211,000 to 95,000.

Platelets allow our blood to clot. When they decline below twenty to forty thousand, hemorrhage can occur. In Damion's case, anything could set off unstoppable internal bleeding. The rubbing of a catheter against an irritated edematous bowel or any other unseen internal stress could start a bleed. A cerebral hemorrhage could also erupt at any time. Damion's life was in danger of bleeding away.

As they came out of the machine, the frequent printouts from the lab were grabbed by Danny and passed to Dr. Cahil, our pediatric hematologist, and Dr. Havis, the pediatric nephrologist. Then Marnix saw them and lastly they were passed to me. The numbers showed rapid platelet destruction. This morning's 6:10 hematology report from the lab read only 20,000. Blood work was increased. Needle after needle penetrated Damion's fingers. People from the lab visited with little round disks of white paper. They stuck his finger and timed how long it took for the bleeding to stop, pressing his pricked finger to the absorbent paper and making a wheel of blood prints. "Twenty minutes," the nurse told me while the disk was still picking up little blots of blood.

"How long does it normally take before bleeding stops?" I asked.

"About two minutes."

The blots still came. The nurse gave up and wrapped a bandage around Damion's finger.

These were the microscopic dangers: shattered platelets, fibrin split products, and shredded red blood cells. This sludge presented its own deadly possibility: coagulation. This trash had already clogged the minute filtering vessels (the glomeruli) of Damion's kidneys and taken them out. Now because blood is the vehicle by which all oxygen and nutrients are carried to our organs, every one of his organs stood vulnerable. Marnix and I locked eyes in mutual misery. "Stroke," "micro emboli," and "infarct" were added to our dreaded vocabulary list.

Upheaval reigned in Damion's blood. It was anyone's guess which organ system would topple next because of this anarchy on the cellular level.

So what were parents to do except stand by and cross our fingers? In the United States, the treatment for H.U.S was to keep the patient alive until the beast in the blood exhausted itself. The treatment was to hope and pray that the beast would not make a fatal "hit" on a major organ. Pick up the slack on damaged organs like kidneys and lungs that we have technology to assist. When the beast retreated, and if the patient survived, "mop up" the damage.

With support as the only response, a patient who was a child could eventually be sent home a diabetic because the pancreas had been ruined. Or sent home needing dialysis the rest of his life. This was how it was: medicine had no other treatment but to allow the disease to run its course. Some children would need only minor assistance while others would be severely damaged, with lives ruined before they had a chance to unfold. Some children did not go home. Damion's dramatic decline in platelets and the rise in fibrin split products made him more likely to fit into the last two categories of victims. Yet we had no better choice. We had to surrender him to a certain fatalism of how H.U.S was managed. But today was also the day of plasma.

On the way back to Damion, I passed Marnix, Dr. Havis, Danny, and Dr. Cahil standing in a circle by the desk.

"What is the down side?" Marnix was asking Dr. Cahil. Marnix held his notepad against his thigh. He strained, listening. He seemed poised for another refusal. He turned to the others and said again, "What's the down side?"

I kept walking and entered Damion's space. Damion and I and a new nurse passed what was left of the morning. Damion was sleepy and barely aware of the intruding needles, dialysis, and a parade of pediatric specialists checking on him. Marnix stayed mostly out at the desk consulting with doctors or made telephone calls from our parent room.

Some phone calls appear to change everything.

Marnix hung up as I entered our room. "There's no time to explain it now, Mary. Damion doesn't need platelets. He needs plasma! I've got to see Danny!"

He slapped his tablet hard against the bed before he rushed out of the room. I could see from his face what he'd heard had galvanized and revitalized him but he didn't have time to talk. Today was the fifth day Damion had gone without food, and by now he was depleted of calories and protein. He could not go on fighting his battle without nutrients. So early this morning Danny had initiated TPN, or total parenteral nutrition. Nutrients were mixed specially for Damion based on his needs based on constantly updated lab reports. The mixture looked like brown soup. It was so refined and sterile that it could be infused directly into Damion's circulatory system through the subclavian line under his collar bone. The TPN dripped slowly around the clock, and every few hours a nurse delivered a huge syringe of albumin into this line to provide him with protein. Complimenting this steady diet was a glass bottle of creamy white lipids, tipped upside down and connected to an adjoining line. The bottle looked like the kind of old-fashioned milk bottle that used to be delivered to our door when I was a little girl. It provided the one homey note in a room full of complicated technological equipment. The cozy appearance of the milk bottle alleviated my worries about keeping Damion fed.

Has anyone ever adequately explained how a mother feels about her children's hunger? I wonder if anyone can understand this unless they are equipped with a mother's instincts. Marnix always seemed blank on this aspect of parenthood. If we traveled or if he was working with the children at lunch time and they missed a regular meal, it drove me crazy. He thought I focused too much on getting the children fed when they were hungry. But I felt my children's hunger. I felt it when they were babies and cried for milk. Theirs was hunger as a kind of pain, and it became my pain as well. Today, a gnawing pain in me was soothed. A visceral panic was calmed by an upside down milk bottle that would keep my boy from starving.

Our new nurse, Pepper, was engrossed in keeping her charts. I offered to read to Damion, but he didn't want me to talk. He was drowsy still, and his eyes flickered now and then as though confusion passed over him. There was an uncertain aspect about him; his statements seemed more tentative now, as though there was a loose connection in the wiring of his brain. Soon he dozed off and left me alone with my sense of wonder at what had happened to our calm lives. How had we landed in this uncertain, chaotic world in which life and death hung by a tenuous thread?

The unique environment of the intensive care unit had its own unspoken rules of protocol and etiquette which we were learning quickly. Most of these rules developed out of respect for the privacy of other families. You didn't look at the other patients or their parents. You kept your eyes fixed within your own glass space.

When you passed another cubicle, you looked only straight ahead. Outside the unit, you usually didn't speak to the other parents. And when you did, it was in careful phrases. It was as though each family's fear and pain were so heavy that to take on another's burden would be overwhelming. Even the professionals adhered to these rules. Nurses didn't make even passing references to other patients in front of other families. This was difficult to achieve in a blatantly exposed environment.

Near us was the cubicle which housed the baby I'd passed last night. Baby Marty was the exception that made us all break the rules. Baby Marty had spent more time in intensive care than anyone else. He'd been there since birth. Now he was seventeen months old. I'd heard the nurses fight about which one he loved the most. His space was opposite Damion's. It was a large glass room with balloons swaying out of his reach above his respirator equipment. With Damion sleeping and Marnix and the doctors momentarily scattered, Pepper invited me to follow her into the baby's room. Pepper was young, blond, athletic, and irreverent. She enjoyed bending the rules a bit.

"He did go home for two days once," Pepper told me. "But he missed us so much he had to come back. Marty has severe pulmonary problems. He has grown up on the respirator. He wasn't supposed to live, but we're showing them!" Pepper glowed with pride.

"Once he really worried us, though," she said. "He pulled the hose out of his tracheotomy, turned blue and arrested. Code 19 all over the place. We had to revive him. He really got it from us when he came to."

She lowered the side of Marty's crib and leaned over to nuzzle his face. His body bounced and he kicked out in delight. "Isn't that right, Marty?" Pepper cooed. "You really got in trouble that day. You know what, fatty? You're getting too fat again. Dr. Plasencia's going to have to cut back on your feedings. Gimme a kiss. Otherwise, I'll tell the doctor how much you weigh."

If you were not disarmed by the baby's smile and the love everyone had for him, it would have been easy to find Marty's appearance shocking. A respirator hose plugged directly into a hole cut into his neck. His head was horribly enlarged from the steroids that he needed. A comic young nurse endearingly nick-named him "Potato Head." Everyone loved and cared for Marty. The friendly respiratory therapist, Robert, would come with a Radio Flyer wagon to take Marty and his respirator for rides around the unit, an adventure which took an hour's planning. Robert would induct a nurse who wasn't so busy to trail a few paces behind push-ing a wheelchair loaded with Marty's ventilator equipment. And, every time she could break away, Jane, another nurse, would play with him, stretch his legs for exercise and spank them with love. Dr. Plasencia would lean over his crib late at night and tell him stories in Spanish.

"Danny's going to be sure that Marty is bilingual before we'll let him go home," Pepper said. The idea of Dr. Plasencia trying to teach a second language to a baby who'd never been able to make a sound struck me as beautifully absurd. It was an example of the kind of hope and dreams that these people had for all the children in their care. I was learning from Pepper and Danny and Terri, all of them, not only how bad it could get, but how a rare honorable goodness can grow from tragedy.

When Marty's mom came to rock him, the nurses partially slid his door closed and tilted his blinds shut. Later I passed by and saw her holding Marty in the oak rocking chair the hospital provid-ed for her. Pepper told me the mother had other small children at home. I never talked to Marty's mom. She came and left without a word. But she taught me a lot about patience. "If she can hang in there for that baby's entire life, I can get through these days with Damion," I told myself.

At the end of the morning, Marnix asked me to come with him to our room.

"Tell me." Now he had time to talk.

"Okay now. This is beyond belief. There is something going on here. A pattern is developing, something profound and even spir-itual is happening. You know how I've struggled with faith and all that . . . but something is happening here. Every time something awful happens, a door opens up for us. This is so unbelievable."

"Tell me about it."

We sat on opposing fold-down beds.

Finally, he could explain. "Thanks for being patient. Okay, when I read that H.U.S. is basically a blood disorder, I thought of an old friend from medical school. He was at the top of our class. We lost touch, but I knew he was becoming a hematologist when I went to Montreal for McGill and he went on to Duke. His name is John Kelton. I heard that he ended up at McMaster."

"Is that who you tried calling yesterday?"

"Right. But he wasn't there. His secretary told me he was out of the country for two weeks. I left a message with his associate. John called in and spent hours trying to track me down. He called Ben, remembering that my brother set up practice in Massachusetts. Anyway, he called everywhere trying to find us. I never left a number for him thinking it was a dead end."

"That's who Liz told me about."

He nodded. "He's chief of medicine at McMaster and directs a lab with lots of researchers doing advanced work on clotting disorders. He knows about H.U.S., Mary. He says what Damion needs is plasma."

"But Dr. Havis said plasma exchange is experimental and unproven," I questioned. "Who do we listen to?"

"We listen to someone who devotes his life to platelet disorders at probably the best center for this in the world," Marnix said.

"What about the dangers of blood transfusion? Do you want to take that on?"

"John says the risks don't compare to the danger Damion's in. If we continue with only dialysis, Damion has a very big chance of dying. His case is severe, incredibly bad by the first indicators. Because he's an older child close to adolescence, he has a more dangerous overlay of T.T.P., which has a very high mortality rate. It's almost always fatal without plasma exchange. If he lives, he'd have a very high likelihood of major damage. There is no debate. As far as I can see, Damion is falling into a deep hole. This is the one hope."

John's the only one with real knowledge of this damn disease; the others are working in the dark.

Something wasn't making sense to me. A disease they saw so seldom. Something so rare, Marnix had difficulty finding articles on it in a medical school library. Something so uncommon that it hardly earned a paragraph in his pediatric texts. Before I could formulate my questions he returned to the urgent topic of what to do now.

"I think Danny agrees with this. He's got no ego involved. He's caught in the middle, acting more or less like a moderator in the decision although I think he's on board conceptually with John. Havis and Cahil have been talked into going along with it. Danny's lining it up for today. A Dr. Finley from the Blood Bank is on the way over."

"If this works . . ."

"It must," Marnix said decisively. "We have someone wise and open in Danny and someone on the cutting edge in John. We'll make it work. We have to."

Marnix went on. "Mary, we have to save him. And just maybe it's beginning to turn our way. Listen to this. The day Damion was admitted, John Kelton began his two-week vacation. All other times, he's so busy that he doesn't have time to take on more cases. And, Mary, guess where he flew the day Damion came here?"

"I don't know," I said wearily. I couldn't grasp all this.

"Where do Canadians like to take spring vacations? Think!" He paused and then answered happily, "Florida. His family's at Delray Beach on the east coast. He's willing to consult by phone or, if he's needed, to come here."

What could I say? I prayed. *Redemption has followed us to Florida.*

Now there was work to be done. Danny needed to put in a line where the plasma could be infused into Damion. This meant cutting down into his femoral artery, so that a line could be threaded in. Parents weren't allowed while procedures like this were done.

"We'll be right back," Marnix promised Damion. "Be tough, animal. You're really doing well today."

Damion seemed not to have heard. As soon as we were in our room I asked, "Marnix, what's this flickering I saw this morning?" I asked, concerned. "Have you noticed Damion's momentary bouts of disorientation? It's not like yesterday's almost poisoned confusion. It's," I paused. "Flickering, for lack of a better word."

"I know." Marnix nodded. "He makes sense one second and then he loses his train of thought."

I pressed. "Is it from all the drugs, or yesterday's anesthesia? Is it still all the toxins that dialysis can't pull off fast enough? It's probably that, isn't it?"

Marnix didn't want to say it, much less believe it. His worry was only conjecture. There was no way to be sure. "Maybe it's one of those reasons, or a combination of them. Or it could be the beginning of something else." He looked away, staring into the distance.

"What? What else? What are you worried about?"

"We're both worried about it," he answered. "Or we wouldn't be having this discussion. Platelets, a clotting disorder. Micro emboli. T.I.A."

"T.I.A.?"

"Transient ischemic attack."

I sighed heavily. "You mean mini-strokes."

"We won't be starting the plasma one minute too soon," he murmured as he got up to see if we could go back to the unit yet.

"One more second, Marnix. I saw this earlier on the dresser. What does it mean?"

"WATCH OUT FOR."

"Watch out for what?" I pointed to the page.

"Pancreatitis," Marnix said quietly. "One fourth of the cases develop pancreatitis."

"Oh. And that would mean?"

His voice was strained. "Ultimately it could mean diabetes."

"I guess we have to do this one step at a time?"

"Right." He looked relieved at not having to contemplate the future. "Right now let's get him hooked up to plasmapheresis."

WEDNESDAY AFTERNOON

So this was it. This was the evil exposed.

"Look how orange it is," Marnix said to me, amazed.

It was a nasty purulent output. I compared it to the straw-colored plasma infusing in the other line. The contrast was dramatic.

"It's so much thicker and cloudier," I said staring.

For two-and-a-half hours we watched the contrast. The machine, the size of a microwave oven, hummed, spun, and exchanged Damion's serum with healthy donor plasma. One at a time the bags of fresh frozen plasma were unpacked from the cooler, two liters all together. Dr. Finley of the Blood Bank told Marnix that was Damion's estimated plasma volume. The plan was to execute a one-to-one exchange. The Blood Bank nurse was too intent on keeping the process going to be able to speak to us. She watched the tubing that fed into the new femoral line cut into Damion's groin. She checked and rechecked the codes on the bags. She adjusted the cycling machine. She recorded everything. She was so engrossed in her job that Marnix and I talked across her.

"Look how orange it is," he said again.

I nodded. The evil toxin remained unnamed. But it was here in the output tubing. It was here, hiding in the destruction it ignited. We could see its angry orange color. It was here in the danger we hoped so much to siphon off.

"It's in there, isn't it?" I said in a hushed tone. Both of us stared transfixed by the sight of the tubing drawing off Damion's ruined blood.

EVENING

In the cafeteria, Marnix stood with Dr. Finley who was giving him an update on today's plasma exchange and the late afternoon lab work.

I searched for a table in a sea of hungry hospital personnel. It was peak hour for dinner. "Marnix," I said, watching his exhausted face. "Sit and eat with me. Here's some salad and some bread. We've both got to eat something."

"John used an apt word in our conversation before," Marnix said as he collapsed in a chair. "He really knows how to put things clearly." Marnix was tired, he was hopeful, he was starving, he was inspired.

"He said that H.U.S. involves multi system damage, and that the destruction unfolds in a sort of domino progression. Here's the word John used: *cascade*. Isn't that just perfect? Doesn't that just wrap up everything that's happened in Damion?"

"Nice word, lousy meaning," I answered.

He nodded. "I don't want to be down here long, but is there soup or something over there? Let me have a few dollars and I'll get some juices too, for later. Be right back."

I considered Dr. Kelton's word, cascade, as Marnix got up. The cash register line was long, and he'd have to wait behind a crowd of people balancing full trays. He was thinner now, I thought as I watched him lean over the glass counters looking for something carbohydrate and filling. This was the first time he'd eaten down here with me. Now I was more nauseated and tired than hungry. All the voices in the dining room flowed into one ribbon of low continuous chatter, like the sound of water babbling over rocks.

Cascade. It was really a beautiful word. It described one of nature's rare surprises. The summer I was Damion's age, my parents took me to Yellowstone Park. I remembered Cascade Falls there. I thought that was what its name was. I remembered the surprise of a river disconnected, a stream abruptly broken, then long plumes of white and glistening water plummeting down. It was beautiful to watch, a beautiful accident of nature when the ground was abruptly pulled out from under the will of that river.

And the falling had assumed an unnatural slowness. The frothy sheets descended so slowly. The water seemed to disobey the rush of gravity. Long bands of displaced water stretched and pulled at the tautness of time until time itself was suspended in a slow fall. It was a beautiful falling down, a beautiful warping of the bands of time and water, a beautiful disregard of the inevitable crash that took place below.

But oh, how the meaning of a word can change! A person with memories of its former beauty could learn its uglier use, hear this word in a new context with grave meaning. In our case, suddenly we found ourselves tossed in the roiling water, victims of a revolting roll over the smoothed precipice. We had felt the earth drop away. As with cascade's other meaning, time was stretched into a protracted plummet, an elongated free fall into danger. Destiny was the fatal rocks below.

Such a word was the one used on the phone to Marnix by Dr. Kelton. Cascade. It could describe a perfectly beautiful anomaly of nature. And it could define the perfect nightmare.

After our dinner I received a message at the P.I.C.U. desk that my father had called. Using the pay phone in the deserted visitors' lounge, I called Washington. Suddenly I felt like a child again.

There was so much to cover to fill him in on, especially since he was a doctor, a brilliant pediatric ophthalmologist. Slowly I related to him Damion's symptoms, the diagnosis, the blood values, the developments. He listened to my long review of all that had happened to Damion over the last four days. He interjected nothing, asked nothing, said nothing in response to each episode of our deepening crisis. And then I stopped. There was a long pause where I momentarily felt like the child who had just placed a broken doll on my father's lap to fix.

He broke my reverie. He asked anxiously, "What's the etiology?"

I didn't know what to answer.

"The etiology," he repeated sharply. "What is it?"

"I don't know what you mean, Dad." I struggled, confused, almost angry that this should be his one and only question.

"Etiology," he repeated again even more slowly, punctuating each syllable. "What's the source, what's the cause, where is the infectious agent? There must be an agent. A child would not go through a dramatic decline like this without some causation. What's the etiology?"

"Nothing's coming back from the lab that can explain. . . ."

"The key is etiology. That's where your answers lay. That's where you'll find the underlying logic of disease progression. That's where you'll find a solution."

During our conversation about Damion's illness, I didn't understand the meaning of his singular question, "What's the etiology?" But over time this question would resonate, and eventually unlock an issue much bigger than Damion, a mission much larger than any I could dream of as I stumbled about on the phone line, not able to help my father with his painful frustration nor answer his incisive question.

As a grandparent, he was distressed about this flagrant attack on his grandchild. As a scientist, he was disturbed about the unexplained reason. While I tensely wound the cord of the pay phone into angry metallic snake coils, he changed direction.

"Your marriage will reach another level," was the only consolation his honesty would allow.

I thought back twenty years ago. Another phone call back

then had told me of how my brother Peter died in my father's arms in my parents' bedroom. I thought of how forever changed my father and mother were after Peter's cancer and death.

"You and Marnix will have a different kind of marriage after this. You will be stronger together."

As I hung up the phone, I knew I didn't have the kind of father who would fix my broken doll. I had the kind of father who would tell me how to fix it myself, and if I couldn't, how to manage the loss.

On the way back to Damion and Marnix, I sucked in my breath. "We'll see, we'll see, we'll see, we'll see. We'll see what becomes of all us three," I recited in rhythm to my footsteps on the hopscotch carpet squares.

Then I pushed on the swinging doors of the P.I.C.U., transitioning from daughter to mother and wife.

WEDNESDAY, LATE EVENING

The printer typed out the blood work from three hours before on the slippery paper. It noted that at that time platelet count was 20,000. The count from thirty minutes ago read, "Platelet count: 14,000. ALERT: LOW."

This number was abstract to me but as I looked first at Danny then at Marnix I saw the fear it caused on their faces.

For a while, this had been a good day. It had been a day of informed decisions and accomplishment and the hope of new plasma. Now it was a bad day again. Actually it was night. It was eight or nine o'clock. Danny wouldn't go home. No one could believe the low numbers from the lab. These were blood values below the danger line of potential hemorrhage.

"If plasmapheresis will work, it has to help soon." Marnix turned to me and spoke ominously. "An improvement has to register soon."

Again, Damion slept. It was the kind of sleep from which he could not easily be roused. It was sleep as a force. It had its own profound power that increasingly overwhelmed him. No one seemed worried by that type of sleep but me. I supposed such sleep was familiar to those who worked with critically ill children. For now Danny and Marnix remained more concern about platelet numbers.

"Marnix, if the platelets are dropping to such extreme levels, why don't you all just give him more? They can give different blood components, can't they? Why not platelets?"

"Yes, they can give platelets. That's the big temptation. It seems like the logical thing to do. But John says it's the worst thing to do. You have to see that the problem is not the platelets themselves—it's the underlying process that is destroying them."

"But why not just give more when there's such danger of hemorrhage?"

"It's like throwing more fuel on the fire. It's adding more fuel that leaves more trash to form more clots to knock out more organs. John tells me the danger from bleeding is far less than that of feeding the beast more platelets. We just have to wait until the beast exhausts itself, and avoid the temptation to do the obvious, like giving platelets. It's a tactical approach, rather than reactive."

Fourteen thousand. Now I understood their dread over this number.

In the dimmed room, it started as a black trickle. Now the nosebleed was so heavy that we had to hold tissues against Damion's sleeping face. I watched his ears. *Please don't bleed, please don't bleed*, I prayed. Marnix was seething in his chair on the other side of the bed. Danny paced back and forth from the fluorescent desk area into our gloomy space. He didn't say a word. I looked to his face for reassurance, but he gave none.

Through my mind raced all the dangerous things that this portended. I visualized other hemorrhages . . . an intestinal one, a cerebral one. I stared at Damion's waxy face.

These could be happening now as you sleep and bleed. But I won't think it. Nor will I look at the red circle blooming on the new tissue that Marnix holds against your nose.

I will look only at your hair, Damion. That's all I will think about, the healthy wisps that sail on this pillow. Baby Damion, your hair is still blond in my fingers. While you're far off, I know that you can hear our thoughts. Listen while Momma tells you this good night story. Listen, Damion, it's about another March, when your baby ringlets bounced white and buoyant as you toddled along.

Daddy is taking us for a Sunday afternoon stroll on the golf course. Most of the time you ride high on his shoulders. But sometimes you get down and shuffle along, scuffing up those ridiculous, hard soled shoes that parents jam onto baby feet. Gravel kicked along the path and baby babbling.

The only words you know are "Mama" and "Da." But on this walk you repeat, "Moo . . . moo." Dad and I kept talking as you waddle behind us.

"Moo . . . moo . . . moo," more insistent now.

"Damion, you sound like a little calf," says Papa, bending down to tie your laces. When he gets down on your level, a lovely crescent is revealed to him, just under the tree tops that hid it from us big people.

"Moo, Da!", you point triumphantly.

"Oh Mamma, he's talking! His first word!"

And we all fall down on the grass, just to laugh and laugh. Our baby can talk! You were seeing something that we could not from our vantage point, and you were telling us about it.

Do you know how powerful you were, Damion? Knocking down grownups on the golf course at eleven months old, making them roll around like fools, laughing until they cry as they passed you back and forth, all just by saying one piece of a word. Damion, that's how strong you still are, baby.

Be tough. Fight this bad thing.

What are you able to see that we cannot?

Please come back and tell us about it.

Finally, after midnight, the nosebleed stopped. Once again, Marnix and I took turns sleeping so that one of us would always be with Damion if he awoke.

9

Hairpin Turns

THURSDAY MORNING, MARCH 5

Marnix had slipped out before I woke up. It was two days after Damion's surgery to implant the catheter and one day after his first plasma exchange. Dialysis was becoming routine. John Kelton was coordinating the team of doctors. I tried to think of the positives, that all of this meant we were doing something about the disease.

But today the beast inside Damion began to rage in another direction. As I pushed open the doors to the unit, I heard a voice on the other side.

"Can you stand back? We're coming out."

A large black machine was being pushed out of the unit by two men with "Radiology" embroidered on their shirts.

"Excuse us, ma'am," they said as the machine rumbled past me toward the elevator. They'd been here for Damion, again. So far, he was the only child in P.I.C.U. that this machine had come to. As I entered the cubicle, I found Marnix standing beside Danny at the illuminated wall. There were three chest films of Damion mounted. Even I could see they showed a progressive cloudiness from the clear area on the left to shadows on the right.

". . . pulmonary edema." I caught the end of Marnix's sentence.

"Yes, good morning," Danny said to me. "Come see this." His face was grave. "I'm afraid there's heart and lung involvement. You can see that there is fluid at the left base of the lung and a slight infiltrate at the right base."

He pointed out the areas for me. I took a deep, trembling breath. It was true. Haziness had started to fill in between Damion's ribs. The "infiltrate," as Danny called it, looked like milky strands floating in the general cloudiness.

"And the heart silhouette is slightly enlarged."

"Yes, definitely, it looks as though someone took the balloon that was his heart and started to inflate it."

Oh my God, I thought.

Danny continued. "We're going to have to do something to help him breathe. I've ordered an echocardiogram and called for a pediatric cardiology consult, Sidney Brodsky. He's very good. You'll be meeting him as soon as he comes in.

"Damion started having difficulty in the early morning hours," Dr. Plasencia continued as we all turned toward Damion's bed. I saw that he was in trouble. He was wide awake and panting as if he had just run a race.

"It's getting hard for you to breathe, Damion, isn't it?" Danny focused on Damion. He brushed aside some of the lines on the mattress and sat on the edge of the bed. Intently, he watched Damion's chest. And he studied the white blinking of the monitor as he rubbed his chin. The oximeter now registered high eighties. I'd learned that it should stay in the 98 to 100 percent range if he was properly oxygenated. Danny pursed his lips, making a decision.

Marnix was rigid, staring at Damion's panting, quick, shallow breathing just as I was. Damion's nostrils flared. His eyes looked wildly from one of us to the other. As though to talk would use too much energy, he whispered to Danny, "How can we make the white number go back up?"

Danny's hand was on the boy's heaving chest. He tried to lighten Damion's anxiety by saying, "Good question, Damion. I see that it's hard for you to breathe. This can make you very tired like you are when jogging all day. We don't want to wear you out. We're going to help you. We're going to move you to a room across the unit. The one straight ahead, where baby Marty is. You'll have more space there. I'm going to put a tube down your throat that will give you more air. That way you won't have to work so hard. It will make you feel much better. Do you have any questions about it?"

"Same idea as a scuba diver. Will Marty be my roommate?"

"No." Danny smiled. "We'll move Marty for a while. Okay, now. One thing that will be different with the tube is that you will not be able to talk. But we'll help you with that."

Danny turned to Terri who was standing in the corner against the sink. "Terri, can you get a communication board from Child Life?"

He talked to Damion again. "You will use your hands to talk with us. And we'll give you a board to communicate with us by pointing."

"Will it hurt?" Damion whispered.

"No, the tube won't hurt. It might feel strange, but it's something that you need now to help you."

Damion's lungs were taking a whack now. This was loop three of the roller coaster ride: colon, kidneys, *lungs*. But, I prayed, *Please look after his brain, God.*

It was time for Marnix and me to leave again. Aside from being in the way, it would only be upsetting to have us there and would complicate Danny's work during the intubation.

In our parent room, Marnix and I agonized.

"Marnix, what should I do? I know you want to stay and be here for Dr. Kelton's calls and can't leave Damion. You want me to go get the van before it gets towed away?"

"Okay. While you're out, you could check on Sebastian. He needs to see us. I know he's very frightened. His voice trembles when we talk to him on the phone, poor boy."

"I don't want to be gone for long. I want to be back within two hours. Listen, I'll check out of our room at the club, get my suitcase, talk to Sebastian, and line up the counselors to get him to the airport on Saturday if we can't take him. Do you agree with me that Sebastian shouldn't come here to see Damion just yet?"

He nodded. "Seeing Damion would be a bad idea. Sebastian's scared enough as it is. And it's all we can do to keep Damion alive. Sebastian can come when we know Damion's getting out of the woods."

"Agreed." I started to gather up my key ring and wallet for the taxi.

Marnix took my hand. "Mary. Damion's getting into deeper trouble. You understand that, don't you?"

I refused to answer. "I'll get a cab," I said.

Marnix persisted. "You need to know that this is bad today. Do you?"

Still I didn't answer. "I'm gone, Marnix." I grabbed my purse and ran away.

Outside, the sunshine glittered as if this day were full of promise instead of foreboding. Cabs were lined up at the hospital entrance. I got inside one and gave the driver the address to Lennox Hospital. So many things were strange now. For instance, this man was probably wondering why I needed a ride from one hospital to another. I wasn't about to explain it as the cabdriver retraced the trip the ambulance made three nights ago. I used the time to think about what to say to Sebastian.

I found the van where I'd left it on that early hazy morning only two days before. It was drenched in sunshine. Heat shimmered off all the cars in the lot and from the pavement. Heat roared out of the van as I unlocked the door.

"I will drown in all this wet heat," I moaned.

But there was no time to waste. I put the key in the ignition and headed the van into the traffic and the big swirling gulf of wet air and space that separated Damion from Sebastian. The asphalt gave off that strange mirage of water on the horizon, the kind of illusion that only heat can paint. Submerged in the currents of sunshine and sadness, I rehearsed what to do next.

"Sebastian, you look good!"

Clean sweat beaded on his neck. His wet hair glistened in the sun. What an understatement I had made. Sebastian didn't look just good—he looked magnificent. I had never fully appreciated the exquisite beauty of the healthy bodies of our children. It was just something I had always expected and felt entitled to. Now I couldn't get over it, sitting on this bench at the edge of the tennis court with the resplendently healthy Sebastian.

"Where'd you get the new shirt?"

I can't believe how strong you are, I thought. *Look how full your thighs are . . . and I always thought you were thin!*

"I won it. Mr. Jaeger said I did the best on our court yesterday."

"Well great, Bombie! It sounds like you're doing great. He's a very good teacher, I hear. At least he did fine with Andrea. You really do look good to me."

Sebastian looked downward. His strong fingers picked at his racquet strings. Another drop of sweat slid off his nose and dripped on his muscular leg. I put my arm around his shoulders. "Bombie, I know you're worried about Damion. This is the first time I could come to talk with you about him. Daddy is with him right now, and he wanted me to come check on you and give you a hug."

"What's wrong with Damion?" Sebastian asked, not looking up at me.

"Well, it's complicated, and I don't understand it very well . . . but D.D. has a problem with his blood and kidneys that is making him very sick."

"Is it an infection?"

"It's like one, I think. The doctors are trying to find out why Damion's blood got so messed up. And they're working very hard to help him."

Sebastian was silent.

"Bombie, you're helping brother, too, by being so grown up and letting us stay with him all this time."

We talked about how Sebastian might have to fly home alone that weekend and about how we would arrange all these things. We found the other academy students. I spoke with Ken who reassured me he was taking good care of Sebastian. Then we hugged each other goodbye.

"Is Damion going to be all right?"

"Oh, Pup, I pray so. Will you pray for brother, too? We'll call you every evening and tell you how he is. Daddy and the doctors are taking very good care of him. I think it's going to be all right."

"I love you, Mama."

"I love you, too. I'll talk to you tonight."

He looked big and strong when I walked away from him. Big and strong and scared.

"I love you, Mama," he bleated after me, a lamb undeterred by the older children on the courts around him.

"Thank you, Bombie. We love you so much, too. You're a special boy. This is going to be all right, okay?" I waved, thumbs up to him as a triumphant signal. It would have been cruel not to lie, leaving him alone like that.

I started the drive back only to find the road clogged with cars. What is going on with this damn traffic, I thought. I idled on the ramp off Route 75 for fifteen minutes. I flipped on the radio to get a traffic report and learned that it was strawberry festival today and President Bush was visiting the area. There were celebrations everywhere in Tampa, except in our hospital where I was supposed to have returned an hour before.

"Great, just great," I muttered. "Now we've even got the President of the United States adding his name to our ever growing list of complications!"

I told myself:

At times like this, one has to resolve not to become angrier. It's pointless to digest your own stomach lining. Crank up the air-conditioning, turn up the radio to the loudest rock on the FM band, inch along behind that bumper ahead. Know that you are powerless. Accept that you are at the mercy of forces you'll never even see. Never forget that, so you don't become surprised when everything gridlocks in your life.

White hands gripping the wheel and my head pounding, I inched forward. Finally, an hour and a half later I arrived at the hospital.

"May I come in to see Damion?" I asked over the phone outside the intensive care unit.

Alice, the benevolent dictator nurse, answered, "Yes, you may." She said this in exactly the tone children use during the game of Mother, May I.

Through the open blinds I saw Marnix sitting close to Damion's bed in the space we took from baby Marty. All around him, the dark room was filled with machinery.

Marnix's back blocked my view of Damion as I approached the sliding doors.

I stopped to gather my courage. What on earth had I expected, I asked myself. Did I think this was going to be a breeze? Did I think a respirator breathing for my boy was going to be just one more complication loaded on top of the rest? One more thing like Tampa's traffic still stalled below Damion's window, or abandoning my other child, or fluid seeping into Damion's lungs and his heart inflating?

Nevertheless, despite my efforts at rationalization, when Marnix's angle changed and I saw my once healthy son, I could not believe it. I propelled myself forward but I could go no further than the foot of Damion's bed. I gasped. Marnix raised his finger to his mouth, "Ssshh." He gestured for me to come in closer.

Damion slept under a tangle of blue ribbed tubes on his chest. Two hoses came together, fused to a smaller hose taped into the corner of his mouth. Surgical tape was taut around his face and circled his head, tightly holding his jaw in a grotesque position. My son was bound by tape locking the tube in place. He was gagged. Creepy pneumatic pumping. He depended on all this machinery with big dials and a pump that forced breath into his lungs.

"That's it," I murmured, half under my breath. "This one I cannot stomach." I pivoted out of the room and hurried past the desk, hand over my mouth. The nurses gave me a look halfway between sympathy and guilt as I rushed past them.

Marnix soon followed me to our parent room.

"There is no way, no way," I cried.

"Come on, Mary. You've got to see this like you do the exchanges, as helping. He needs it."

"I know that, but there's no way I can stand this."

As if anyone was offering me a choice of whether I could stand it or not. This was a lesson I had yet to grasp. I was still learning. We are not allowed to choose how much we can tolerate. And what a place to learn it. An existential hell.

AFTERNOON

There was no plasma today. Damion was not in good enough condition, it was decided. At three, the pediatric cardiologist joined the team. Dr. Brodsky was looking over the echocardiogram that Danny had ordered and was studying the mounted x-rays that now were five in number. He looked about the same height as Danny as they stood together behind the desk area. But as dramatic and chiseled as Danny's features were, Dr. Brodsky's were bland and mundane. His hair was sandy brown and his manner was low-key, distant, maybe even shy. Dr. Brodsky's height was medium, his build was medium, his coloring was medium, everything about the way he moved was medium.

His manner was completely serious as he came in to see Damion. He gave us a cursory nod. I offered him my chair beside the bed but he gently pushed it out of the way so he could lean over the sleeping Damion. Brodsky listened to Damion's chest for a few moments, then slowly draped his stethoscope across his shoulders.

He began to speak to both of us. "My impression is that he does have pericardial effusion as well as fluid accumulating in his lungs. We need remove the fluid that is accumulating around his heart"

"When?" I asked.

"Now."

"Is it done under anesthesia?" I asked. "Does he have to be put under general?"

"We'll give Damion something that will make him drop off momentarily," said Danny. "It will take the edge off, but he will be awake."

"A needle right up against a beating heart. How can you manage to keep it exactly at the place you need to?" I asked, trying not to visualize a slip-up.

"We'll see clearly, guided by the echocardiogram. We control that."

"Do you need to do this downstairs in the OR?"

"No, we'll do it here. He stays right in his bed."

Danny finished up the meeting. "We'll come to your room and let you know as soon as it's done. That should be in thirty to forty minutes." This meant it was time for us to go and wait outside again. Marnix and I thanked them and got up to leave. On the way out, Marnix bent over to put his face up to Damion's hair. I laid my hand on his foot. Both of us managed to do this carefully. Damion didn't awake. As we stepped into the hallway, we saw the mobile echocardiography machine coming off the elevator.

What do you do while someone inserts a five-inch needle into your child's chest to try and save his drowning heart? Marnix and I had no idea. We sat on my bed side by side, facing the door. I leaned over, my elbows on my knees, my hands locked under my face. He was doing the same. If one of the St. Joseph's nuns came into our room at that moment, she would have been pleased to think we were both praying. Marnix might have been praying, but I was not. I was absolutely numb, too numb for words. Prayer would have taken too much effort, or at least presence of mind. Waiting for a report on what happened as they stabbed Damion's chest and tried not to nick his heart, I had nothing left with which to pray.

Marnix was perhaps in the same unplugged condition. Neither of us had an impulse to say a word to the other. We sat under the seemingly unmoving clock. We sat and sat and sat.

Finally, the door opened and we jumped up as Danny and Dr. Brodsky came in. Four people stood around my bed. For the first time since we'd come back there, my words returned. "Please tell us something good," I whispered.

Danny spoke.

"Damion tolerated the procedure well."

Then Dr. Brodsky reported.

"I drew off three hundred and fifty-five ccs of fluid, nearly a liter. It was a surprising amount. More than I had anticipated." He paused, then continued.

"Thank you, Dr. Brodsky. Thank you very much. Thank you both," I said.

Marnix and I shook their hands and they departed. We felt a little better. At least the fluid was out. It was probably the same weeping fluid that was seeping everywhere now from Damion's damaged vessels. Chest tubes would drain the fluid from his lungs. Damion's heart was rescued! Roller coaster loop four now: colon, kidneys, lungs, and heart, and we still hadn't fallen out.

"But you know what I don't understand, Marnix? If this is such great news, why is Brodsky still so grave?"

"Maybe it's just his manner," Marnix answered hopefully. Hope was what we needed. I took his statement at face value and didn't probe.

"Yes, he does seem like a very serious man," I replied.

Marnix and I sat beside Damion as he slept deeply through the evening. I tried not to look at the quarter-inch tubes now puncturing his chest from Danny's efforts a couple of inches down from his nipples. They looped out of taped holes. Under his bed the clear plastic container where the fluids were collecting was just as offensive. The fluid, a syrupy red-tinged runoff wound its way down the tubes and coursed into the already surprisingly full bags. I wondered if Marnix had the same response to this new system that I had: a mixture of horror and relief. Horror at how drastic it looked. Relief that all this drowning fluid could now drain off.

The respirator breathed methodically; the monitors showed steady numbers whenever we looked up at it. I leaned on Damion's bed and watched the monitor, the only moving thing in the room besides the ventilator. The numbers held steady and hypnotic. As I watched, they fluctuated only a few points, showing the kind of slight variation that resulted simply from being alive. But then, in an instant, an aberration occurred.

"Marnix, look!"

The systolic and diastolic numbers on the blood pressure monitor started to dance.

Surely I imagined that!

But I had to know. I pointed to the screen.

The numbers flickered between normal and low values for a second, then steadied.

"Just an inconsistent reading, don't you think that's what it was, Marnix?"

Marnix glared at the monitor.

Suddenly it jiggled again. The digital display started spinning like the window of a slot machine. Strange numbers, this time longer than for just a second.

110 over 40.

80 over 45.

85 over 40.

"What the hell!" Marnix cried out.

Instantly the alarm screamed both here and at the desk. Two nurses hurried to Damion's side. One ran back to get on the phone. We stood frozen. Damion began shaking. The nurse punched numbers into the monitor. No one said a word.

60 over 35.

The other nurse came running back holding a syringe. Damion's face was ashen.

50 over 30.

Trembling turned into convulsing. Now his face vibrated blue. His arms flailed wildly on the mattress.

"COME ON! COME ON!" somebody shouted.

40 over 20.

Marnix grabbed my arm and piloted me out of the room. At the door I saw the nurse pumping the syringe into Damion's IV line. The other nurse drove the crash cart into Damion's room.

"We can't be in there now, Mary. Come on," Marnix growled, his grip hurting me.

Uniformed men we'd never seen before ran into the room as Marnix pulled me out of the unit.

"Oh, God, please. Please God. Please, please. Please God, please." That was all there was left to whisper as we leaned against the wall and each other outside the unit door. You don't know what begging is until you pray to God to let your child survive one more minute. That was all I asked for.

Marnix went back in and returned to the hallway to get me. "Damion's blood pressure is climbing and steadying. He isn't shaking anymore," he reported.

"How much did he need?" Marnix asked the nurse who stood near one of the IV bags.

"Danny's on his way over," she answered noncommittally.

The uniformed men left quietly. All the rest of us stood in silent guard of the monitor. Damion was far, far away from us.

He had almost wandered off too far this time to ever return.

A stillness fell. Quiet, unexpected, yet profound. I questioned the silence:

Was it professional restraint, everyone performing their jobs with perfect dignity under pressure? No, this was not merely the quiet of competence.

Was it fear? No, it was more intense.

Was it suspense? No, that was a cheap explanation.

Later, I figured it out. I knew what the stillness was as we waited for Damion to return. Death was a frequent visitor there. Sometimes Death beckoned a child out of the unit. Sometimes He sat beside a crib or bed and only laid his hand on a little forehead. Everyone here submitted to His presence. All paid silent homage to His final authority. He was the stillness I heard.

It was after midnight. I felt a responsibility to transmit positive feelings and thoughts to Damion. It didn't matter if he was in a deep sleep, or even a state close to coma. In fact, that's when it became more important than ever for me to send him strong, confident thoughts. Although this may sound foolish or mystical, I know that it mattered and that this was what I was supposed to do while others tended to his numbers and values.

So I pulled the chair up against the bed, put my head beside his on the pillow and listened to his slow breathing. The respirator noises, the blips and bleeps of the IV pumps and monitors faded. It was just us again. Memories and thoughts leapt the synapse between us. His vulnerability and proximity to death made him somehow receptive. How did I know this? I don't know how, but I did, and so will you if you ever sit beside your child fighting for his life.

It's just you and me again, boy. Precious Damion, do you remember two months ago? You and I couldn't believe the cold!

"How do you know that minus 34.4 degrees Celsius equals 30 degrees below zero?" I had asked.

"Mrs. Danner taught us the metric system. Zero equals 32 degrees Fahrenheit. So figure it out, Mom. Minus 34.4 is 30 degrees below zero Fahrenheit."

"So, that's why they use metric up here in Canada! Minus 34.4 sounds a bit warmer than 30 degrees below zero. If they told people how cold it really is, all these Québécois would move to Alabama."

"Mom," you moaned, rolling your eyes.

"It's not supposed to be this cold in the daytime. But that can't scare us away, can it, D.?" I hold your poles with mine against my side. They're tucked in under my elbow so I can sit on both hands, like you. Our breath comes out as vapor through the ice crystals that grow on our knit collars. We pull our turtlenecks up to our eyes.

"Sacre bleu, monsieur Damion! Look at dis! A waterfall of ice! And voila. . . . Can you see zee weather station on

Mount Tremblant?" You ignore me so well when I act like a jerk. . . .

Beautiful cold. Beautiful glistening snow. Windless air so cold that it can make conifers pop. The sound of skis slicing through snow, amplified by the cold.

"Damion, aren't we extremely lucky to be above all of this?"

You give me a polite nod. You are busy watching for the end of the lift and planning the next step. "You follow me this time," you say as you pull up on the bar.

"Okay, big boy. You're the boss, as usual."

For someone who skis reasonably well, you move like an awkward giraffe getting off the ski lift. You know that's the reason I hold on to your poles until you gain your balance at the end of the steep dismount ramp. Otherwise you'd wave them around wildly and would tangle us both up. Once we slide out of the lift's way on the icy bulge of the mountain top, it's time to straighten out our gear.

"All right, Mr. Bond. Goggles on, buckles snapped, here are your poles back, James, sir. Parachute checked, engines on . . . let's fly!" And that's what we did. Over and over, all afternoon. You ahead of me, your tracks smooth and sinuous on the slopes. Just you and I and the cold and speed. Wasn't that one of the greatest days ever?

10

Seesawing in Space

Friday, Saturday, and Sunday. All these days clot into one memory. We went from begging for each hour, back to praying for each day. Damion did well. Damion did poorly. But he stayed with us. No more wandering off.

Every day, Dr. Finley and a nurse from the blood bank brought the equipment and plasma. Eight to ten bags of beautiful, viscous serum were laid out on the bed, tagged, numbered and rechecked three times against the master list before the exchange was made. It was meticulous work, requiring full concentration by the nurse as the machine cycled and replaced Damion's own toxin-ruined plasma.

Please work. Please work. Please work.

The machine's rhythmic whine infused hope into this plea of ours.

When Damion awakened, Marnix and I tried to entertain and engage him. But he was awake so little. He could manage to stay up for perhaps thirty minutes and then he sank back into deep sleep. He had no interest in television. He found the book I tried to read him irritating. I drew cartoons on his communication board at which he wouldn't laugh.

But Damion remained responsive to Dr. Plasencia. He would eagerly communicate with him by writing feeble notes whenever Danny came in to check on him, which was almost hourly. Much of the communication between them had to do with a pact they made:

the respirator would stay only until it wasn't absolutely necessary, and Damion could try to drink fluids as soon as he was weaned from it. Damion fixated on Danny's goal of removing the "breathing tube" on Wednesday. The two of them talked a lot about what Damion could drink then.

It was a wonder to me that the fine, wirelike line Danny had threaded into a vein beneath Damion's collar bone could carry all the nutrients he needed. I knew what it took to keep this boy fed: volumes of cereal, platefuls of french fries, and these were just his snacks. By now, it had been an entire week since he had eaten his last meal of pizza. It had been one week since he drank soda or juice. For his strength and resources to be maintained, the IV fluid and the orange bag of TPN became critical components of his care. Amazingly to me, hunger didn't seem to pose a problem to him.

But thirst remained a powerful urge, judging by the number of questions he strenuously scrawled to Danny about the targeted day midweek.

"And I can even have a Slurpy? My mom can go to a Seven Eleven and bring it to me. Strawberry."

"Do they have any Sprite downstairs?"

"Will it be the first thing you do on Wednesday?"

"When you take it out, can Terri have two cups of ice water ready?"

For now we could only moisten his mouth with glycerin sticks, keep Vaseline smeared on his lips, and be grateful that sleep shielded him from so much of his want. But then the thought occurred to me that dreams are often ways for us to work through our frustrations. It made me sick to think that his were probably about fluids.

On Friday afternoon, on my way back to Damion's room, I passed Danny standing with an attractive woman.

"This is my wife, Nilda," Danny said proudly, then darted away to another child in the unit who needed him. Nilda was lovely, very soft spoken, with large soft eyes. She, too, was of Latin origin.

"Danny's been telling me about your family. It must be so hard to have a sick child. I can't imagine what it would be like. I'm sorry you are going through this."

I asked her about her three children, two girls and a boy. I lamented that Danny couldn't be home more with them, but thanked her for all the time he'd given to us this past five days.

"Nilda, your husband's been so wonderful. There would never be a way for us to thank him for what he's doing. No matter what happens to our boy, I'll always know we got the best care imaginable for him."

FRIDAY EVENING, MARCH 6

Marnix and Dr. Kelton had a lengthy telephone conversation that expanded beyond the moment-by-moment crisis management they had focused on until then. Marnix talked with me afterwards in the deserted parent lounge.

The new location was a good space to broaden our horizons, literally. It was perched on top of the building eight floors up and had one large glass wall that overlooked the city. Now at twilight we could see the nearby oval of a stadium, the cluster of tall buildings downtown, the airport that Marnix came into, and Tampa Bay which always gave this cityscape a soft and hazy glow. The city seemed so beautiful, yet so indifferent to one boy struggling within it.

Marnix talked about his broadened understanding of Damion's case. John's experience and information had added new layers of insight this evening.

"You know that Damion's age has been an important factor in all this?"

"Why?" I asked.

"Because he's an older child, the likelihood of complications beyond the initial kidney failure is increased. H.U.S. is a global disease because the damage happens through the blood. That's why it threatens every organ of the body. Often times, the older a child is, the rougher the ride," Marnix explained.

"Then it's a bad thing that Damion has this happening to him now instead of when he was three or four?"

"In a way, yes. He has an overlay of the disease T.T.P. on top of his H.U.S."

"Even when the disease is recognized, the treatment for H.U.S. does not usually include plasmapheresis. Damion's getting plasma exchange only because he's older, and because John understood the T.T.P. connection. In that way we're lucky about his age."

Looking down at the busy traffic on the avenue below, I had the dizzying sensation that the holes in information and the advancement of care were not what all us non-medical people expected. The image of the doctor descending into the bowels of the hospital to go online to other centers worldwide, scanning for the latest, most aggressive therapies, the way it was in movies, was false. This was the stuff that television advertisements for pharmaceutical companies were made of. The thought was maddening to me.

"Don't get me wrong, plasma exchange is not a magic bullet that will automatically save every child. But it's the most potent and logical therapy at this time. Some of the children who are dying don't have to. And many who survive with major damage would have less damage if they got plasma exchange on time, frequently enough and for long enough."

"Kids are dying who don't have to be dying," I said, incredulous. "All because there is an unfinished argument between nephrology and hematology? So, why don't parents know this?"

"Two reasons: number one, there's no one who has gotten the funding and multi-center backing to organize all these cases into a study to prove on a wide scale basis the scope of this disease and the benefits of plasma exchange. Number two, Politics. Some influential physicians are turf protective."

"So, what do they tell parents?"

"They say, if they are typical, 'This disease has no treatment and no cure.' They say, if confronted about plasma exchange, 'I'm sorry, it's not been absolutely proven for H.U.S., and it's too risky.'"

"It's true that it can be dangerous, especially in the days of AIDS." I hated to think about this. I repressed the thought whenever I saw the bags of plasma laid out on Damion's blanket. Marnix knew my fears, and was good enough always to say something emphatic like, "Here they are Mary: pure, fresh frozen healthy human plasma. . . ."

Marnix debunked this excuse about risk. "But these are the same doctors that have no reservations about throwing platelets or packed red cells at a critically ill child. Any blood product carries a risk of transmittable disease, platelets more so than plasma. And look at the numbers of this, and the reality of it, too. Without exchange, in cases with T.T.P. involvement, the risk of dying is substantial and the chance of lifelong severe physical impairment without exchange is maybe as high as seventy-five percent.

"With exchange, the chance of contracting hepatitis B, which you can immediately immunize for, is minimal. The chance of Hepatitis C is maybe one in thirty. The chance of contracting H.I.V. is one in a couple hundred thousand. If you're looking at a child whose chance of dying is one in ten, to one in four in nasty cases, the least a physician can do is to offer any hopeful therapy as an option to that child's parents. But that's rarely what happens."

"We need to get this medical information out to families," I said emphatically.

"I agree. Most families are totally dependent on their doctor and his approach. And you see how it is, Mary. Do you think that if I were anything else in life, a carpenter or a business man, that it would occur to me to call specialists all over the world to get their opinions? It wouldn't even be an option to go to a medical library and pull up articles and be able to understand them. Even if I wanted to do so, there's no time with this disease. Once the roller coaster ride begins, you're on it twenty-four hours a day reacting from one emergency to the next. You think we'd be able to take the time to investigate?"

"No. It would be impossible," I murmured.

"And there's another obstacle. People need to believe in their doctor. It's an essential human need almost. When all hell breaks loose, and you don't know anything about this big, complicated world of medicine, and you need that world more than anything to keep your child alive, you are naturally going to invest all your belief and hope in that one professional standing between your child and death."

"Yeah," I agreed, thinking of the immediate bond we forged with Danny. *Now* I was even more depressed over the unfairness that all trusts in doctors were not so well placed as ours. Our good fortune in accessing knowledge and care made the misfortune of others all the more unacceptable to me.

"So you really mean to tell me, Marnix, that some kids who wouldn't have to die are dying, because of professional ego? That if

Damion fell into the hands of such a specialist, he'd have been dead by now and we'd never have known that there was more we could have done to try and save him?"

Marnix's answer was an indirect yes. "Doctors are human."

For all the parents that would never know, I felt very angry.

As the darkness ate the last bit of sky over the Gulf of Mexico, I interjected, "There's only one thing to say. As Damion would say, that sucks." Frustrated, I was worrying over the entire forest, while Marnix was wise enough to fight for our one little sapling.

FRIDAY NIGHT

Tonight, Damion was stable enough for us to try and go to bed at the same time. Everything was quiet and steady in the unit. Danny had gone home hours ago. A new nurse had been assigned to Damion for the night shift, Saracita. Sara, as the other nurses called her, was a very beautiful blend of Black and Spanish, whose accent told us she had been in Florida for many years. She was careful, competent, experienced. I had seen her work over the critically ill little baby in the tented crib the last few nights. I noticed her intensity with her charting and yet her gentleness with the baby, the way she adjusted its lines and tubes and rubbed its wrinkled little back.

So Marnix and I felt we could get one night of sleep together.

"Marnix?" There was nothing between us but a huge gulf of silence and darkness. Our bed units were fastened to the wall as far apart as the room allowed with a wide dresser positioned between them.

"Marnix, you awake?"

Marnix has the habit of listening with an earphone to CNN News all night as he sleeps. I don't understand how he can stand the constant stimulation. I always teased him that it was going to short-circuit his neurons, but he was content to sleep this way. I realized that with his earphone in one ear and a pillow over the other, he couldn't hear me from across the room.

I missed talking at night. With our four children, night had been the only time of day that we had been able to talk for years. So I crossed the great divide of our room.

"Can you just hold me a minute?" I knelt beside him.

He pulled me onto his narrow cot. Like two spoons, we managed to fit by lying side to side, my back to his front. This was how we always fit so well together: him wrapping around me.

"We haven't been able to go to bed at the same time since this started. Even though we're together all the time, there's so much we have to concentrate on. Are you too tired to talk a minute?"

"What is it?" His breath was warm on my neck.

"The Florida Boards. Neither of us understood the real motivation for you to prepare for them, especially me. I'm sorry I fought you on it. I'm sorry I didn't trust you to do the best thing for our family."

He grunted, then rubbed my back, massaging me gently.

"This is the real Florida exam. This is why you had to study and review all you had forgotten. This is the real test, isn't it?"

Somehow, we had begun to rock gently.

"Marnix, is he going to live?"

"Oh, we're trying everything, everything to help him."

"I know. I know. I just have to know so I can get ready if he doesn't." My tears dampened his arm propped under my head.

"Both of us have to get ready for anything. He's got John, he's got Danny, he's in a very good hospital. He's getting more of a chance than almost any other child with H.U.S.." He sighed. "We have to be grateful.

"Very grateful," he repeated in the moist dark space behind my neck. He paused and, as if he spoke to himself as well, said, "And pray."

That was why I loved my husband, I thought to myself as we almost rocked to sleep.

Despite his hopeful words to me that night, Marnix became very quiet over the next few days. He was mulling over the meaning of T.T.P. added on top of Damion's H.U.S.

Thrombotic Thrombocytopenic Purpura was bad news. Extremely bad. John had told Marnix the numbers, but Marnix failed to report them to me. T.T.P. entailed more complications to major organs. T.T.P. came with a steeper price tag, as diseases went. It had a higher fatality rate, an extreme mortality of up to

90 percent in one study of patients who didn't receive plasma-pheresis.

SATURDAY MORNING

We found Danny in the unit very early. He was sitting beside an associate of Dr. Havis whom we'd seen very briefly one evening before. Her name was Sharon Perlman.

Dr. Perlman was shaking her head, sitting at the desk next to Danny who was writing. Her white lab coat had several pens tucked neatly into her breast pocket. She uncapped one and made two small circles on a page. When Marnix leaned over the counter of the desk from our side, she handed this lab report to him. "These are his worst numbers yet. Last night Damion's BUN was ninety, and his creatinine two-point-two. This has truly been a renal insult for Damion. The dialysis helps him hold his own, but we have to be very concerned about these numbers as they continue to elevate. We'll just have to see if there is residual damage when they come down."

The possibility of permanent renal damage was something Marnix and I had talked about. Hypertension might result. Or worse, the kidneys wouldn't fully turn back on, and Damion would face hemodialysis.

"These children don't grow or thrive as well. They don't have a life, hooked up to machines." Marnix said.

Then there was the worst possibility of all for Damion's kidneys: end stage renal failure. "He'd be on a long list for organ recipients. And he'd be facing not only the trauma of transplantation, but would have to be on all sorts of immune suppressants to walk him through the hurdles of rejection. That would be a terrible thing for him to face."

"If his kidneys do not resume their function, if Damion has permanent impairment, what will we do?" I tried to imagine our active son with a life that had been pruned back dramatically.

"We'll deal with it. First let's focus on getting him through the disease. The kidneys are a big worry, but they're just one concern," Marnix answered.

His response, "We'll deal with it" reflected a kind of prayer we both secretly prayed:

*We'll take him home with kidney damage. We'll take
him home with pancreatic destruction, a diabetic if that's
what has to happen. We'll take him home with lung or cardiac impairment. We'll take him home with a colostomy.
We'll take him home neurologically damaged. Blind or
stroke damaged if he has to be. We'll deal with any of that.
Please, please just let us take him home.*

Since Thursday, the cardiac complication had reinflated, until it now threatened to explode. Danny asked us to follow him from Damion's bedside to a new series of chest x-rays that had just come back up from Radiology. They hung on the wall, suspended by small clips that fastened them over the lighted panels. The films showed Damion's heart dramatically enlarging, more than the x-ray from last night. Now it hung heavy in his chest like an engorged water balloon.

"This concerns me." Danny traced around the edges of Damion's heart with his index finger. "Looks like pleural effusion as well. We're going to have to do something about this now."

"Are we looking at another pericardiocentesis?" Marnix asked.

"I want to take another echocardiogram and have Dr. Brodsky decide if there is any effect yet of this fluid on myocardial functioning. Let's see what he says."

We returned to Damion as Danny picked up the phone. Our door was open and we couldn't help but strain to hear.

"Yes, good morning. This is Dr. Plasencia. I need another echocardiogram on my patient Heersink, Damion. No, as soon as possible, yes. Emergency basis. Yes."

By 11:30 A.M., Dr. Brodsky was interpreting his findings for Marnix behind the unit desk area. To me it felt like an instant replay of Thursday's conversation with the same participants of Danny, the pediatric cardiologist, Marnix and I. We stood near the identical props: chest x-rays and echocardiogram tracings. And here again was that unchanged sober demeanor of the always serious Dr. Brodsky. "The fluid seems to be about the same amount as yesterday's reac-cumulation. I'd say a moderate to large amount. We're about where he was on Thursday, only now with more heart enlargement."

"I gather that this puts Damion in even graver cardiac danger than he was on Thursday," I said. "Because not only has the fluid reaccumulated to the same degree within his pericardial membrane, but the stress of this fluid is now beginning to negatively impact on his heart function. Doesn't this, on top of his right lung filling up with fluid, add another layer of danger?"

"Yes, that's about it." Dr. Brodsky nodded at my unschooled attempt to summarize what he'd just laid out.

"I don't think we can avoid it. I'm going to have to do another pericardial tap."

There are lots of truisms about marriage. Most of them have been honed over the millennia by men and women living together, trying to resolve their conflicting natures and forging a marital unit that withstands the bruises of life. The key to a good marriage is to not only make your two personalities fit together in some kind of delicate truce, but to allow them to complement one another, to chemically bind one person's negatives to a partner's positives, one person's abundances to the other's deficits.

For example, one of the cliche little bits of advice that actually turned out to be a solid rule was given to us both upon marriage by Marnix's dad. Opa was a towering figure in Marnix's life, a powerful authority. "Never go to sleep still angry with one another," he lectured us at our wedding reception. It was a good thing, because in the dark inner spaces of night your partner's slights and selfishness can assume monstrous proportions. If you go to sleep disliking each other, you can wake up hating one another.

The challenge of Damion's illness demanded that we improvise new rules within our marriage for handling this extreme stress. These were never articulated. We never hashed the rules out. But somehow these laws naturally developed, and they made certain times bearable that otherwise could have torn us apart with grief.

One very important code that governed the balancing act of dealing with Damion's disease was, "Never both believe at the same time that he will die." At all times one of us stood guard over the fragile hope that Damion could keep on being rescued from one threat after another. Usually, one of us was submerged in fatalism and despair while the other acted as a buoy, anchoring the other to the surface with a thin line of hope.

This was not a contrived arrangement. We didn't sit over cafeteria coffee and decide which one of us was going to delude ourselves for the day's incredible struggle. This division of hope wasn't assigned according to who had the most sleep or who knew the most or least about medicine, or who pulled the most weight of believing over the last few hours or days. It wasn't determined by logic. It was absolutely unpredictable which one of us would believe on a certain day. Rather, it became an organic response that grew out of the innermost needs of our relationship. And unlike the "Never go to sleep angry" rule, which we'd broken maybe five or six times, we never violated this new unspoken rule, *Never both think he's going to die.*

Both of us had crushing fears and loss of faith. Both of us were scared to death of what was likely to be the outcome. But we could never let ourselves have these emotions at the same time. And so, without consciously deciding it, we simply took turns.

This week, and more particularly since John Kelton's involvement, Marnix was the strong one for me. He bridged my lack of knowledge of the doctors' expertise. He was my interpreter in this foreign and dangerous land. He excavated a treatment option in the form of John's guidance. He negotiated a speedy implementation of a new therapy. He laid out for me the grand design of the game plan. Marnix was the positive directing force. For this brief but intense period, he was the keeper of the timid flame of hope. I relied on his light, but because of this he trod the darkness alone.

When I came back into our parent room in mid-afternoon, I found him curled away from me on his bed. I had wondered where he'd slipped off to. A nap? This was an amazing time for a rest, with Dr. Brodsky about to do another pericardiocentesis. Sitting down on my mattress, I considered what we should be doing while Dr. Brodsky performed the second pericardial tap.

Tap. What a word. As if this was early March in Vermont and the woods were thawing on sunny days, the sap was running, and Damion was a maple sapling. And it was syrup boiling time, time to hang the buckets and hammer in the taps. God, I thought, I'm getting tired. We're all getting tired. I rubbed my forehead and tried to shake off my growing distraction. Then a sound penetrated the silence. I looked across the room to see Marnix's shoulders shaking as if he was crying. Was he crying? I tiptoed over to his bedside and knelt down beside him.

"Are you okay?"

His face was buried in his hands and his neck was very red. I felt mystified about what to do because I hardly ever saw tears other than a few happy ones over our newborns' screaming in the delivery room. Tears of grief had overcome him only after his father's grueling death.

"I'm here, Darling," I said, enveloping him.

He continued to weep as I rocked him.

"This is just like my father," Marnix said. "Days and days of watching him deteriorate. Everything going wrong. Pulling him out of one hospital where they were going to let him die, moving him by ambulance to Nijmegen, lining up surgeons, fighting to get him better care, opening him back up again, getting more powerful antibiotics set up for him, all for nothing. Failing. One catastrophe after another as everything shut down. Days and days of watching him die of a stupid infection. An infection, for Christ's sake! A bad belly. It was unbelievable, an unbelievable clumsy death.

"And here we are in a replay, this time with my own son. It's all happening just the same way. Our boy is dying a stupid, stupid death from an infection, from a bad belly. And once again there's nothing I can do to stop it."

"No, no," I consoled. "It will work this time." I rocked him again. "This time it will all work out. It will, it will, I promise. You are saving Damion. John is saving him. Everyone here is rescuing him. This time it will work. Everything will be good again. Everything will work."

I wasn't just saying these words. It wasn't just to comfort him and not believe them myself. Because on this seesaw of believing, the amazing thing was that when Marnix went down, I really did go up. To me, at this hour, on this afternoon, Damion was going to make it.

11

Moments in Isolation

THE NEXT HOUR, fear set in again. When they were ready to take the second pericardiocentesis, Danny asked us where we'd be. When we hesitated and shrugged as though we couldn't think what to do with ourselves, he suggested, "It will take about an hour. Why don't you get out and walk or something? Get some fresh air and come back at four, okay?"

It was easier obeying than coming up with a plan ourselves. We got into the elevator, exited in the cool marbled lobby, and wandered down a ramp into the awful heat of afternoon. We walked on a sidewalk that had tufts of centipede growing through the cracks. The sidewalk ended and we crossed Martin Luther King Boulevard. There was a megalithic mall in front of us, rising out of the steamy asphalt. We saw stores such as Sears, Burdine's, and Ruby Tuesday's and followed the procession of people to the entrance. Most had their children with them. Inside, we were surrounded by mannequins in exaggerated poses, sun care products, florid perfume, and young women behind makeup counters wearing orchid eye shadow. Escaping this hothouse atmosphere, we walked to a sun-drenched atrium and found a food court.

"Let me buy you an orange juice," Marnix said.

We stood against a stand that squeezed orange juice in a big, plexiglass machine. A young man took Marnix's change and handed over a frothy, cold drink. We sat at an ironwork table and placed the orange juice between us. We didn't really drink it. We just took turns sipping so we'd feel we had reason to be there. Marnix's eyes were red. My throat was on fire.

"Let's go back now," I said after ten minutes. We got up and threw the remainder of our drink in a trash bin and wound our way past all the redundant and universal franchises that make American shopping so predictable: Radio Shack, The Limited, Waldenbooks.

A true cross-section of Florida humanity strolled up and down the mall with us. *These people* did not include the sunburnt tourists; that crowd remained on the beaches. These people all looked to be resident Floridians.

There were body builders in muscle-man shirts going into the General Nutrition Center. There were young mothers trailing little children in cartooned T-shirts. There were sparkly overweight older women in hand-painted sequined creations that seemed to erupt without warning on this year's fashion scene. If the plan was to have this boisterous knitwear distract from their growing girth, it wasn't working. But they did look effervescent, especially with their stiff bouffant hairdos.

The most fascinating groups to watch were the teenage girls in bare midriff tank tops. They collected around The Gap and Victoria's Secret, twittering and darting like long-legged sand-pipers. They looked around nervously with birdlike head movements as they scanned everyone outside their circle. They were saying "Is he looking at me?" and "Those two are cute" as we shuffled past them.

I looked longingly at the people at our stage of life. Men with collared knit shirts and women in sleeveless pastel dresses shopping with healthy girls or boys in Michael Jordan Nike gear. They sauntered along in confidence, so sure that all was well in their world. Even though they resembled us in age and fashion, I felt isolated as though we had suddenly and irrevocably severed our ties from normalcy.

All these people in the Sunday afternoon mall, all these subtypes and age groups across the socioeconomic spectrum were dizzyingly happy, just as we had once been, only they didn't know it.

We returned to the burning pavement. "Oh, Marnix, all that was so foreign. We don't belong there anymore with normal people. I don't know if we'll ever belong anywhere again," I said.

Marnix just squeezed my hand tighter. We retraced our steps to the hospital, took the elevator to the eighth floor, and arrived at the unit a few minutes before four.

"Wait here a sec," Marnix said. "I'll see if they're through."
He pushed on the wooden door, peered around it, and signaled for
me to come on. Danny and Dr. Brodsky were behind the desk leaning over a gray paper with tracings of Damion's heart.

"Come in," Danny said.

Dr. Brodsky leaned toward us.

"Same thing as two days ago," he said. "This time I drew off
three hundred and seventy-five ccs of a slightly opaque yellow fluid
that showed no evidence of blood. His follow-up echocardiogram
shows a small amount of residual fluid, but I see no apparent fibrinous exudate in the pericardial fluid I couldn't reach during the tap."

Dr. Brodsky brightened, giving us as much as he was capable
of hopefulness. "We are still getting 'No Growth' reports from
Bacteriology on Thursday's tap. Let's hope today is the same situation. Maybe the infiltrate in his right lung will start to clear," Danny
said. "I went ahead and inserted another chest tube to drain this
while he was mildly sedated for the tap."

Danny looked at us. "Now let's hope all this effusion stops."

Please, God. Please again.

SATURDAY EVENING

Our family life had been relegated to phone calls during
which we all tried to connect.

Marnix talked to Sebastian about his plane trip back home.
There was a lot to do for a ten-year-old. "Okay, pup, tell me again
what time the limo's going to pick you up? And how long do you need
to pack the things that aren't already in your bag? Yeah, but give yourself enough time to double-check around the apartment, okay? The
driver knows what part of the airport to take you to. That's all worked
out. He's going to walk you into the terminal and take you to the
check-in desk. You don't have to worry about a ticket, because it's
going to be there waiting for you. And don't worry if the man or lady
at the desk says you need your parent's signature for you to fly. We
already worked that out on the phone, and it's on the computer, tell
them. So, all you have to do is check your big sports bag. They'll connect you with an attendant who will get you to the gate and help you
get on the plane. You've seen how children flying alone get all this
special attention, so you know already a little bit of what to expect.

"When you land in Atlanta, it will be the same thing. No big deal, because an attendant will go with you on the train to another terminal for the Delta Connection, just like we always do. You won't be alone from the time you get in the limo until you walk off the plane in Dothan. And then you'll see Liz. Okay, big man?

"Yes, all right you can drink Coke. I'll make this a special exception." I smiled to overhear that this was Sebastian's big concern. Marnix went on to tell Sebastian again that Damion was hanging in there, and that everyone was working really hard to make him better.

"Good night, Bomber. I hope you sleep well tonight. And tomorrow's supposed to be a good day for flying, so maybe you'll see a lot out your window. I love you. Good night, Sebastian." Marnix put the phone down.

"Mary," he said, turning to me, "sometimes I worry about him. Sebastian internalizes everything. He has a hard time letting his feelings out."

Nodding, I smiled at the insight, wondering if in part Marnix was speaking of himself, too.

I felt a need to talk with someone who knew Damion, someone who knew him for what he was before he became this desperate boy attached to machines. I called a friend who drove him to school as a kindergartner and laughed at his repertoire of sound effects in the backseat of her car each morning. She was astonished, and promised to help fill my void at home.

And Mrs. Roberts, Damion's teacher. She would have to know as Monday drew nearer. She would expect him at his desk. She knew Damion. She knew his potential and his beauty. She expressed her frustration.

"How can this have happened?" she asked, amazed and sad.

Then the phone call Marnix and I had dreaded most had to be made. It was Saturday night and our youngest children expected us home the next day. Slowly I dialed my own home. "Bayne, it's Mama," I said when he answered the phone. "I have to tell you that we won't be back home tomorrow. Damion is sick and we have to stay down here in Tampa with him. We don't know for how long."

"Can't you bring Damion home to get better?" Bayne asked with the clarity of nine-year-old logic.

"I'm afraid not, puppy. He's in a special hospital that can help very sick children. We don't have that kind in Dothan."

Liz, our baby-sitter, told me later that night that both Bayne and Mila had cried after my talk with them. "But, Mrs. Heersink, don't you worry about these children. You know I'll treat them like they were my own."

"I know, Liz. I've never needed you more. We'll just have to ask you to do everything until we know what's going to happen here. I know Bayne and Mila are in good hands. Kiss them for us."

Marnix made calls as well, including calls to his office manager Frank in Birmingham for help in rescheduling patients. Marnix was running his office long distance on a day by day basis; he couldn't leave us until Damion's heart-lung situation was stabilized. Monday's and Tuesday's books would have to be cleared. Secretaries needed to come in on Sunday morning and start calling the fifty or so patients for each day. Surgeries needed to be canceled. There was no telling when all these displaced people, on top of this past week's backlog, would be rescheduled. But Frank, who traveled to Dothan three days a week to help Marnix, was doing a great job of holding down the fort.

Marnix also checked in with John Kelton to give him another status report. However, the puzzling question John raised juxtaposed perfectly with the unanswerable one my father had posed to me earlier.

"So when did he eat the hamburger meat?"

Marnix shared this question with me, almost reluctantly. It was too much for him to deal with at the moment, and he knew me well enough to suspect it would drive me crazy.

"Excuse me?" was my exasperated reply. "Hamburger meat?"

I scowled at my husband. "This makes no sense at all. Marnix, we don't ever buy hamburger meat. And Damion didn't have any fast food that week except a cheese pizza at Matt Hall's house. We had no opportunity. I can remember every time I took the kids for a special treat of fast food, and we've had no reason or time to do that for at least two weeks. That makes no sense at all."

"John says look back four to eight days from the day he became symptomatic. That's where you'd find what sparked this.

That will establish the time frame of infection."

"Well, then let's culture! Damion's still having extremely bloody diarrhea. Let's ask Danny to broaden the stool cultures! Let's check and see what shows up. Whatever it was, it'll still be there."

Marnix tapped his pen against his notes and shook his head, no.

"John says it's too late for that. Damion's system has already thrown it off. It wouldn't show up on culture anymore. There's often a very small window of opportunity that exists to find this pathogen, and it's usually one or two days after a kid is sick enough to need medical attention. By now, Damion's intestinal tract has thrown it off. The bug has done its damage and left. Its toxins have ignited this whole disease."

Thoughts whirled in my mind. Hamburger meat? Bacteria in Damion's food could have ignited all this? It was impossible. The implications were too impossible to consider. They would require too much of my energy that right now had to be directed toward keeping Damion alive. At that moment, I had no energy to spare for anger, curiosity, or investigation. Who had time to work on a jigsaw puzzle when Damion was fighting to stay alive?

But I asked again, "Hamburger? Impossible. Isn't it the USDA that inspects meat? Remember all the federal inspectors in those filmstrips they showed in high school home ec. classes? Oh forget it, you didn't take Home Ec., and you grew up in Canada anyway. But really, in the States, every meat packing plant has federal inspectors, not plant personnel, but government inspectors for disease and dirt. No, *really*, the more I think about it, contaminated meat has to be impossible."

Marnix reluctantly handed me one more piece of the puzzle. "Do you know that in Canada the provincial government of Quebec, for one, refers to hemolytic uremic syndrome as 'Hamburger Disease?'"

SUNDAY MORNING, MARCH 8

In seven days God created the earth. In seven days Damion's disease had disassembled our lives and recreated them into a nightmare. On the seventh day, God was pleased with His creation, and

He rested. On his seventh day in the hospital, Damion was exhausted by a week of unrelenting physical destruction, and he slept.

Yesterday's second procedure to drain the fluid pooling around his heart had exhausted him. Both chest tubes drained off a serous fluid that Marnix said was the same consistency and color that puddled around his heart. It was alarming to see how much oozed out of him. Now, I could envision what they meant by the term, "congestive heart failure." If this weren't spilling off or aspirated through Dr. Brodsky's needle, it was easy to see that Damion would have drowned in his own weeping fluids.

"Where is all this coming from?" I asked, indenting a clear bag under his bed that was turgid with the reddish runoff.

"It's from the lining of his vessels that have broken down. It's collecting everywhere now. If you look at the x-rays of his lower abdomen, you see it bloating the layers of the membrane lining of his intestines. It's an insidious process. It's all this same fluid pooling in other organs, the same fluid you see in these tubes coming out of his chest."

AFTERNOON

I was alone with Damion when he woke up briefly. He seemed as though he wanted to say something so I gave him the nurse's pad to write on. I cringed to see his struggle to write. The letters were becoming very small, very concentrated, and almost illegible. I tried not to think of it as a reflection of what was happening to him internally, but isn't that what penmanship is? A mirror of the internal person?

I had to prop another pillow under his head to get the angle right for him to see the tablet as he wrote. *"When they put that needle in my chest, it feels like they are STABBING ME!! Why can't they knock me out? It makes my shoulder hurt so much! Even more than my heart."*

I hugged him as best I could. "Damion, I thought they gave you something to make you fall asleep so you couldn't feel it."

Damion motioned insistently for the tablet in my hands, then wrote, "It works only in the beginning. Then I wake up. I can't move. They tell me to hold still till it's over. I try not to cry but they are stabbing me."

"Oh, D.D. I think that's the last time they have to do that. Yesterday they got a lot of fluid from around your heart. This will make you better much faster. I'm so sorry it hurt you."

Damion turned his head away from me so I wouldn't see. I knew he was crying.

Despite my lack of energy to consider what had made Damion ill, I could not rid myself of the question. I asked Danny about the source of Damion's illness when I saw he had a free moment at the desk. "You don't think it could be meat, do you?"

Danny shook his head. "The disease was started by some infectious agent. It was likely something he was exposed to through eating. But there'd probably be no way now to trace it back and determine the exact cause of infection."

"But you cultured his stool for everything; the other hospital cultured it, too."

"Yes, we searched for all the standard pathogens that our labs are set up to look for: shigella, salmonella, campylobacter, listeria, yersinia and vibrio. Those reports are negative. I had an infectious disease specialist in to look at Damion and review his chart. We didn't come up with anything specific."

"But there was something? He was infected by eating? It was foodborne?"

"Yes, most likely."

"And Dr. Marinelli told me that gastrographs of Damion's colon showed thumb printing. He said these x-rays looked as though someone had smeared them with thumb prints, like finger painted thumbs all over his gastrograph. That's unusual and probably means something, too, don't you think?"

I knew that Danny was not a medical detective. His job was to save Damion, and he was using his considerable intelligence and training to get Damion past the critical point. No one had resources to pursue the issue of what the infectious agent was. I couldn't ask Damion about it. He was sleeping nearly all the time now under his respirator hoses, and he was absent from us when he awoke. Marnix and I wouldn't burden him with this worry. He needed every reserve for the fight. We didn't want him to carry one extra concern while every cell in his body was exerting itself in the huge effort to stay alive. We never questioned him about the issue of how he got sick, or said anything to him about our suspicions.

With no ready clues, I dropped it for the time being.

We met Terri in the hallway dressed in street clothes. It took a second before I recognized her. We were so accustomed to seeing her in the same blue scrubs that all the intensive care nurses wore in the P.I.C.U. She looked fresh and attractive in a white sleeveless dress and dangling loop earrings and with her waist length hair falling loose. She grabbed both of my hands. "How's Damion doing since my break began when Friday's shift ended and Saracita took over?" she asked.

She listened as I told her about the second tap, another chest tube inserted, the cardiac enlargement, and how Damion's transient confusion had been replaced with an endless sleepiness.

"I checked on him a minute ago, when I went in to pick up something I'd forgotten. He's hanging in there. He's hanging on." Terri hesitated. She seemed to want to say more to us. And then she got her nerve up to say it.

"On Wednesday night, when he started to get into trouble with his breathing, I didn't think he would make it."

She hesitated again as her eyes began to tear, but then forced herself to say what she felt she needed to tell us. "I did something I've never done. When my shift ended and I finished my charting, I stayed around a few more hours just to watch him. I don't know why I couldn't go home. And then, I went down to the chapel to pray. You see, I watch over a lot of critical kids. This isn't new to me or anything. It's just that I see how much you love him, and I think of my eleven-year-old and how much I love him. I don't know what it is, but I think eleven years is a long time to spend with someone, and then to lose them."

I looked hard at Terri who was always in so much control inside the unit and saw the hard time she was having outside the wooden doors.

"You don't have to explain it. I know what you mean," I said.

Marnix, who had been a silent listener to this up to now, added quietly, "You don't know what it means to us that you are so devoted to him. Damion feels it too. It means a lot to him, and it means so much to us. It's been a big help."

She hugged Marnix and patted his back, then did the same to me. After we took a few minutes to collect ourselves, she regained her cheerful self. "Okay, see you guys on Tuesday. I've got a break till then. You keep everything stable in there, and I'll be back soon. Tell him I peeked in at him while he was napping and that I miss him. And you guys hang in there, too," she added as she backed into the elevator. She waved goodbye as the doors bounced closed.

I turned to Marnix. "How can she do this kind of job and get so involved with her patients? I mean, after a while, this could destroy you if you cared too much."

"What makes her good is that she does care so much," he said quietly.

SUNDAY AFTERNOON

I trudged back to Damion's space.

"Damion, I want you to meet another doctor," Danny was saying. "This is Dr. Sastry. He works with me up here in the unit and watches over the children when I go away. Dr. Sastry will be watching over you starting the middle of this coming week for a few days while I am gone. He's going to look around now and get to know you and catch up with your situation. You'll see him coming and going until Tuesday when I take a short vacation. Then he'll be here for you as I've been."

Dr. Sastry stood in the doorway. He was about the same age as Danny, the same age come to think of it as all Damion's doctors, early to mid forties. That's a comforting age, generally speaking, I thought to myself. Old enough to have a track record of experience, yet young enough to be recently trained. Dr. Sastry had to be good if Danny trusted him, and he seemed pleasant enough. In fact, he seemed quite affable, maybe even jolly. I noticed the way the nurses teased and were relaxed around him.

Danny sat down again on the edge of Damion's bed. He lifted Damion's taped wrists to check the IV lines and patted Damion's upper arm, about the only place any of us could touch Damion now without disrupting a line or hurting him. I loved the way Danny scanned his patient. He looked at all the lines and drainage tubes, the amount of TPN left in the bag, and the color of spent dialysate and chest fluid and urine in bags that lay on the floor or were clipped to the side of the bed. He adjusted the ventilator tube as it pressed against Damion's mouth, as if he was worried about the same thing that bothered me, the discomfort caused by leaving anything in one position too long. Danny seemed to do all this instinctively and automatically. He was attentive, meticulous, and something more. It was hard to define what that more was comprised of, but I thought it had something to do with being a true healer. Danny was someone who had a refined sense of what wasn't already apparent, someone who used his eyes and sense of touch, someone who carefully considered and reconsidered all the details. Danny cared. He immersed himself in a patient's needs and status. His radar caught problems before they came into view. He picked up things others would probably miss because he involved himself so deeply.

Seeing Dr. Sastry standing in the doorway, literally on the threshold of taking over Damion's care, I thought, perhaps unfairly, how lucky we'd been that Damion had landed in Danny's hands. Danny's scheduled rotation in the unit had begun just as Damion came to St. Joseph's. For nine days we were privileged to have his uninterrupted devotion. Dr. Sastry would be fine, no doubt, but I thanked God we'd had Danny so long. Although I'd come to understand why a doctor or nurse had to get away and decompress now and then from a job like this, I couldn't help feeling anxiety about his leaving on that Tuesday.

He sat on Damion's bed.

"But our deal is on?" Damion scribbled to him.

"Yes, of course. Wednesday's the day. If everything goes well and your lungs are ready, Dr. Sastry will take the tube out just like you and I planned."

To us, Danny explained, "I'm not going on vacation yet. I'll still be here through tomorrow. I just want you to become familiarized with Dr. Sastry and him with Damion."

"Thank you. It's very nice to meet you, Dr. Sastry," Marnix said as he shook the doctor's dark and leathery hand.

"Yes, yes." His round head bobbed pleasantly. "I'll look forward to working with Damion," he said in an Indian speech pattern.

SATURDAY NIGHT

> *When did he have the hamburger meat?*

John Kelton's question continued to percolate in my mind. It disturbed me greatly because, first of all, I didn't buy hamburger meat for the children. We shied away from eating red meat out of health concerns about high cholesterol and certain cancers.

Secondly, I was sure Damion had no occasion to be in a fast food restaurant the week before he became sick. It had been a typically busy week. He had soccer practice two afternoons, a piano lesson one afternoon, and a Boy Scout meeting one evening. All the children had busy schedules, and we were always juggling two or three extracurricular activities. Every afternoon was a blur of driving them somewhere. Their after school commitments involved a tactical effort to get each child delivered on time to various lessons, practices, and games that often were scheduled simultaneously. The last thing we had time for during our breakneck afternoons was stopping for a snack. Moreover, Marnix was a strict traditionalist about sitting down as a family to dinner every night. Fast food did not fit into our agenda. I always prepared our dinners while the children were at school. I stored them in the refrigerator so that I could just warm everything up when everyone was finally home again.

There had been no class trips that week for the sixth grade. Sometimes when the children were taken to a concert or to the museum, the class would stop at a food court or a fast food restaurant for lunch. I thought back. No, there had been none of that. That week was very straightforward and ordinary.

As Marnix and I were settling down after midnight in our room, I asked across the dark space, "Marnix, what was the incubation time you told me about?"

"John said it's a longer incubation period than most foodborne illnesses. Think back five, six, seven days before he got sick and you'll find the occasion when he got it."

I continued to review. That was the weekend of Bayne's birthday party. We didn't eat anything diff—

"Oh God," I cried in the darkness. "That's it."

I sat straight up frozen by the realization of what had probably injured Damion. The feeling was like the jolt one must have on walking into a courthouse and confronting the criminal guilty of assaulting one's child. In that electric instant, pictures flashed through my mind of Damion leaving on the Scout camping trip. I could picture the yellow school bus leaving the parking lot with the paper bag containing the meat in the back window. I remembered my fleeting thought about where the cooler was. I also remembered picking Damion up after the trip and his ebullience as he told me about it. While we unpacked the damp clothes from his backpack, Damion told me that the campfire food was so good that he'd eaten four big, juicy hamburgers.

"What's it?" Marnix asked from his corner.

"The camping trip. It was the weekend before when Damion went camping."

I said slowly to my husband, "The Scouts had hamburgers."

12

Humpty-Dumpty

Most of Sunday night I tossed restlessly as the hamburger question revolved in my mind. Finally I gave up trying to sleep and went to sit by Damion for a couple of hours. But eventually I became tired enough to go back to bed. Now Marnix and I were doing what we did every morning, racing to brush our teeth, straighten our beds, and go to Damion before the doctors made their rounds.

After sitting with Damion, there was a phone call I felt compelled to make. I had to talk to Damion's scoutmaster. I had to try to find out where the meat had come from that had made my child so ill.

"Hi, Butch, may I speak with your father? This is Damion's mom." In the background breakfast dishes clattered amid other sounds of getting ready for school, sounds that made me homesick for what used to be our own simple lives. "John, listen, sorry to bother you before work, but we have a serious problem. Damion's in a hospital in Tampa. It's bad; he's in intensive care. John, some of the boys might hear about Damion at school today, and I wanted you to hear about him from us." John was speechless as I sketched out for him what had happened over the last week.

"How could this have happened?" he asked. "I don't understand it."

"That's another reason I'm calling. I think it was from the meat the boys ate on the camping trip, and I'm worried about the other kids."

John didn't say a word, so I went right on.

"We've found out it was the right timing as far as when he could have been infected. And the hamburgers from the cookout were the only meat he had all week, besides chicken."

"Oh my God."

I knew John was astonished and probably felt awful.

"John, listen. No one did anything wrong. It's not your fault, the boys' fault, or anyone's fault who handled the food. If it's from the cookout, then it's an accident. No one is responsible."

For a split second I thought of the government men in the white lab coats turning the sides of beef, and the meat packers who were supposed to maintain sanitation standards.

"John, I swear this isn't anybody's fault. I just need to find out how Damion became sick, and if it was the meat. It's important to be sure none of the other kids got it."

"I haven't heard of anyone turning sick, but I'll ask around today," he said softly.

"John, do you understand how I feel? If Damion got sick from the hamburgers, then this is just like an accident happened, and no one did anything wrong to make it happen."

But it was no use. I had just made a kind, generous man feel miserable. John was shocked enough to hear about Damion fighting for his life. Now to think his Boy Scout troop might be somehow involved was just too much. He was devastated. As we hung up, I felt awful for him.

"Oh Christ Almighty, Mary," I said to myself.

But I had to try to piece together the rough edges of this puzzle and figure out what had happened to my child. I remembered my father's words. "That's where you'll find solutions, too," he had said.

I didn't wish to hurt anyone in order to find the solution. But I would. John was the first one I hurt.

EARLY MONDAY AFTERNOON

Now in his fifth day on the life-supporting ventilator, Damion mercifully continued to sleep most of his hours away. If we added up the moments he was awake, they probably amounted to two or three hours a day. When he did emerge from the cocoon of sleep, he was irritable and disjointed. He didn't want to watch television, which he had yet to watch since being hospitalized. He was annoyed if I tried to read to him, and he was so weak that he could handle conversation in only the sketchiest of ways. Talking with him was reduced to his abrupt pencilings on the notepad and our simple responses and comments to him. Everything about him and his interaction with the world seemed to be limited, distant, receding.

"I know one thing that might pick him up," I whispered to Marnix over the droning and incessant respirator sounds. "A portable CD player. He wants one for his birthday, but I haven't promised to get it for him. I thought I might if he'd pitch in some of his savings toward it."

Damion needed something to connect him to the world, something to bridge the space between the nether world in which he now dwelt and our own, an escape from the oppressive cadence of complex machinery through which hoses forced loud air into his wet lungs. I knew I could find a CD player at the mall Marnix and I had walked to yesterday. I knew, too, what Damion's favorite CDs looked like, although not their album names or even the names of the groups. "I think his favorite CD has a naked baby on the cover swimming after a dollar bill. Nirvana, I think. So that will be easy to find."

So off I went on my well-defined mission. I was in and out of the mall in less than a half hour and back in Damion's room.

"Here, you find a spot on the power strip to plug it in, Marnix. I don't want to be the one responsible for shorting out his IV pumps or other equipment loaded on it. I'll get the cellophane off this. He's going to flip, absolutely flip over this."

When Damion woke up, Marnix placed his fingers on the controls. "Look what your mom picked up for you, D. This is the volume dial. Here's On/Off. This one does Fast Forward/Rewind. I hope you like it, darling. Mom will help you with the earphones." Once they were adjusted, he pushed On. I lifted one of the ear pads away from his ear.

"Do you like it, D.?" He faintly smiled and nodded. But after half a song, his bony hand reached up onto his chest, and trembling along the controls, found the Off button. Still without opening his eyes, he slid the black square off his chest and placed it beside the dormant television remote control below the corner of his pillow.

I sighed.

"It's all right, Mary. He's just very tired," Marnix said when he saw that Damion had fallen asleep again.

LATE MONDAY AFTERNOON

In the hazy late afternoon light that entered Damion's window, I sat with him. It was one of his awake but uninterested periods. Danny came in and pulled up the chair Marnix generally sat in. Dr. Plasencia was quiet, just watching and thinking, until the pictures caught his eye that I had found in the bottom of my purse and taped in Damion's line of vision. They were not fantastic photos, only ones I happened to pick up from the camera shop the day before we came to Florida. There was one of our new German Shepherd puppies, one of us in our kitchen, and one of Damion playing with a soccer ball. I thought the photos might help him focus on his real world of home and pets and sports and school. Danny unstuck the soccer photo and held it in his hand. "Damion, did I tell you that I played soccer when I was your age in Cuba? Yes, I was a very good player, one of the best in my province. I loved it very much, but then I couldn't play any more."

"Why not?" I asked.

"Well, when Fidel Castro took over my country, his army was very angry at my grandfather who was one of the richest landowners in the region, because he was brave enough to stand up to the revolution. My grandfather was thrown in jail, and they stripped him of all his land. His son, my father, was persecuted by the police. Then they wouldn't let me play soccer anymore because I was the grandson of a resister."

Damion's eyes widened at the injustice of it all.

"Then my parents realized that I had to be sent away from Cuba if I was to have any chance of an education or freedom, because the crackdown was making life very difficult and very dangerous for my family. They got me out on the last KLM Royal Dutch Airline flight from Cuba."

"Danny, this is awful. Where did you go?"

"My family sent me to Spain. I was fifteen years old. I then went on to the United States, where I stayed with my uncle. I was very lonely for my home and for my parents and friends and school, but I had to study and work very hard. I managed to get my parents out just before Castro slammed the last doors shut."

Damion listened, seemingly transfixed by the story of Danny's struggle.

"I had a hard time communicating in the United States, so I went to Spain for medical school. Years later I rejoined my family here and studied pediatric critical care. Finally, we're all together in a free country."

Damion's lashes fluttered a second, which they did when he inputted and processed something important. This was the first conversation in days that penetrated the layers of his physical pain. It was precisely what he needed to hear: the story of a young boy who was abruptly ripped from his world. It was the inspiration of that boy's suffering and perseverance and eventual victory that impressed him. The fact that the boy was the young Dr. Plasencia made it all the more relevant. It was the history of the man Damion entrusted his own suffering to.

It was the story of a boy who lived in exile, like Damion now. Its message said to him, *Damion, Damion, you are not alone.*

MONDAY EVENING

The mobile echocardiography machine seemed to be in competition with the portable x-ray machine that thundered through Damion's days. The fact that we could stand there and see into the inner sanctum of Damion's troubled heart was amazing to me. How did medicine proceed before all these window technologies allowed physicians to peer into their patients non-invasively? Was there far more guesswork back then? I thought about all the children with the same disease Damion had who perished before dialysis was introduced and the patients with silent heart disease who died before echocardiography.

"Okay, this is the two-D scanner portion," the blond technician said to Marnix. "I'm going to do several different views. But look, you can see here," she continued, pointing, "the reaccumulation of fluid. How much did you say his last pericardiocentesis drew off? Well, I can't tell if this is that much, but it is a significant amount." But then the technician seemed to check herself and added, "Dr. Brodsky will be able to estimate how much when he reviews this."

121

To me, most of it looked like a confusing mass of pulsating tissue.

"But you do see at least the hint of mitral insufficiency?" Marnix was trying to assume his most dispassionate tone for her, but I could feel the stress in his question.

Perhaps she picked it up, too. "We'll have to ask Dr. Brodsky about that, Dr. Heersink," she said curtly.

Marnix continued to watch the screen, biting the corner of his lip. He asked no more questions. The technician volunteered no more information as she scrolled through several more angles. Finally, as she packed up, Marnix spoke. "Thank you. Sorry we had to get you up here so late in the evening," he said.

"That's what I'm here for," she pleasantly responded to him, now unchallenged.

Marnix motioned to me with his eyes to follow him.

"Good night. Thank you," I said as we left.

In the confines of our parents' room, I asked, "What was that all about?"

"It's playing the game. God Almighty, it's hard. I have to be a dad only, because she won't, in fact she can't, interact with me as a doctor."

"But that's how it goes with all these people, Marnix, except with Danny and the subspecialists."

"That's not what's wrong, Mary. Yes, it's frustrating, but that's not it."

"Well then, what is? Why are you being so intense and upset?"

"Because he's in trouble. Did you see that echo?" he snapped almost accusingly.

"It looked just as confusing and just as shitty as the other ones from my perspective," I said, angry that I was being drawn into his anger.

I should have backed off right there sensing that there was a fireball right around the corner which had nothing to do with Marnix and me, that this was something between Damion and the disease, and something between Marnix and his own frustration of knowing too much.

"You shouldn't curse."

"Why not? I don't see any children in here. And it was shitty, wasn't it?" I said defiantly.

Both of us bristled with anger that was dangerously undefined. Both of us continued to stand, rather than make our way to a chair or bed to sit on. In the slightest movement of compromise, Marnix did, however, lean one elbow against our wall.

"Yes, it was bad. I'm not a cardiologist, and I couldn't begin to understand the nuances of it all, but he's in trouble again. It's not just the fluid that keeps coming back as fast as they can drain it, but now we're probably getting into some damage. This on top of this evening's chest x-ray of his heart being so grossly enlarged—"

"So, what can we do?"

His amorphous anger momentarily retreated into distress.

"He just can't keep on going with this constant pericardial effusion. It's going to . . . well, rather it's already starting to damage—"

"Well, call somebody," I snapped. "Call Brodsky. Ask Sastry to come back in."

Marnix exploded. Something I just said ignited the fuse. He blasted me, more incensed than he had ever been in our whole life together.

"What makes you think you can just demand people to snap into place for us? What makes you think you have the right to act so demanding in this, that everyone will just drop their lives and come running to us? Where did you get this imperial attitude?"

I hesitated, blinded by the heat of his outburst. I staggered, filled with retorts I could have shot back at him. Okay, maybe I was guilty of thinking things could be fixed. Maybe I was demanding a lot from others, but I didn't deserve the full force of this fury at our helplessness.

"You don't understand what I'm saying," I said with angry tears. "I am not acting imperially. If Damion's having a bigger problem and there are people that can help him out of it, I'm not going to apologize for asking for their help, especially when it's their job."

"You don't understand!" he fired back at me. "You can't

snap your fingers and get people at your side instantly. You can't treat people like machines. You think everything can be fixed. You think everything can just keep falling into place for you."

"That's not fair! It's not for me, you idiot! It's for Damion!" I felt guilty as I said this—we'd never called each other names before.

Marnix turned and left the room, closing the door firmly behind him. I furiously stripped off my clothes, threw them at the mirror, and jumped in the shower. "Why are we fighting?" I cried out and turned the water full force on myself. "We're not even fighting about the same thing. He never even heard what I said. He's not even fighting in the same language! This is asinine!"

After scrubbing my hair vigorously, almost violently, I slumped onto the tile floor and wept as I watched the seething water circle into the drain. "Oh God, I just want to go home," I said to myself. "What's happened to everything? Damion is dying and Marnix is attacking me for something I didn't do. God, I'm sick of my throat always hurting for all of us. When will this end? When can we just go home?"

LATE MONDAY NIGHT

Danny was off his rotation now and wouldn't be back for days. No one had called Dr. Sastry. But Dr. Brodsky would be back early in the morning. Damion was sleeping. I watched mesmerized as the chest tubes drained the volumes of sticky tinted fluid into the bag on the floor under his bed. The respirator breathed regularly for him. His heart rate and blood pressure numbers were stable. "The numbers are okay. They are in the safety zone. He's hanging in there," I kept repeating to myself.

Finally, at 1:30 a.m. the nurse turned to us. "You might as well get some sleep," she said, looking first at Marnix, then at me. She probably felt the creepy tension between us.

After lying in bed a long time unable to sleep, I called across the room, "You totally misinterpreted what I said about getting help, Marnix. You don't understand what I'm saying."

"You don't understand what I'm saying," he answered, his anger resolute.

After a long and sweaty pause, I ventured, "Well, since neither of us understands what the other is saying, can we just stop this long enough to fall asleep? I don't know where all this came from, but it's not helping anything."

He said nothing.

"I love you anyway, Marnix Heersink."

"Okay. And I love you. We'll try again tomorrow," he said wearily.

I heard him roll over, then fumble around with his radio and earphones in the dark. I'll never understand, I thought, how two people who have such inseparable bonds in their lives and deeply love each other, can sometimes be so far apart.

TUESDAY MORNING, MARCH 10

I don't know what happened to our argument. I'm not sure either of us figured it out. If you asked at the time or after an interval of years what it actually was about, I'm not sure we could say. Certainly, each of us would say it was about different things than the other would say. The truth remains a large mystery to me, to this day. But it did hurt, and it still makes my throat tight when I think about it. It was the most vehement fight we'd ever had, and it came at the worst and most unexpected of times. How strange that this was our quintessential argument, and neither of us can even agree what it was about.

Maybe it was just about being tired and scared and frustrated, I thought wearily as we put on our shoes that morning.

"Friends?" I asked as we left our room.

He took my hand tenderly in his for the short distance between our door and the P.I.C.U.

Anyway, we dropped it.

At the desk we found Dr. Sastry and Dr. Brodsky. Marnix joined them while I went in to see Damion.

"Good morning, sweet boy." I bent down to kiss him. "Hi, Jane. How are you today?"

Jane was Damion's prettiest nurse. Her porcelain face and her sense of style managed to rise above the same baggy scrubs. If Damion and Sebastian had seen Jane out on the street with her striking features and bluntly cut blond hair, they would have looked a long time at her. Neither would say anything, their nascent pubescence not yet self-aware.

I liked her for her sweetness.

"Hey, Mom," she beamed. "We're just about to strip this bed and get a bath. You want to help?"

Of course I did. Bathing Damion was one of the small pleasures I got every day. It made me feel like I was doing something for him, too. The plastic pan of soapy water smelled like the same soap I used when I used to bathe him as a baby.

Jane staked out the areas of the chest and abdomen, making sure the dressings over the chest tube, subclavian and femoral line wounds didn't get wet. The patches of gauze and surgical tape got changed frequently to avoid infection. I got the arms and legs, one at a time, and then put lotion on his skin because it was becoming dry and flaking. We let Damion wash himself where he needed privacy under his sheet. Then we pulled lines out of his way and rolled him to one side to wash his back and bottom. Now the sheets and towels we'd mounded under him were damp so we undid one corner of the bed, unclamped some of the monitor wires and tubes on that side, positioned the respirator hoses so he wouldn't roll onto them, and scrolled the old linens under them. Immediately, we put on a clean fitted sheet on this corner of the mattress so that when we rolled him over the lump of dirty laundry we could in the same motion pull the clean sheet under him.

"All right, Roly-Poly, that's one side. Now we'll roll you this way and get the other side changed."

The wet linens were wadded into a big lump that I carried to the bin in the central area of the unit, while Jane pulled clean underpants up to where he could reach them. A hospital gown would cover too much of what the doctors and nurses needed to see. And scrub pants didn't work because the blood bank needed daily access to the femoral line portal that was threaded into the top of his thigh.

Jane finished the bed with a top sheet and thinly woven cotton blanket that somehow she arranged into a crisply tailored fold. I had tried unsuccessfully to copy this before and ended up with an unstructured and lumpy bed. The neatly finished covers became one of those little details that gave the impression of order and control to a bed that was otherwise a chaos of wires and plastic tubes.

"Ooh, D., you look dashing." I rummaged in the plastic bin called the "patient care kit" that sat atop a metal cart to see if there was anything else we could do for him. The toothbrush and mouthwash were useless while the respirator tube was taped into his mouth. But I found a small spray can of lemon scent and spritzed it around the room. Then I pulled out the comb and made a part in his damp hair. Jane put a towel over his new pillow case until his hair dried.

Then Jane stepped out to get something. Manning the dialysis machine was a full-time job in itself. Add to that the medications, IV bags, TPN, the respirator hoses, and measuring and emptying the urinary and chest fluid bags and it was easy to see how Damion's nurses were kept on the go all day. Jane would be gone for twenty minutes to round up supplies, knowing that I was with him.

"Your hair is getting so long, baby," I told Damion. "You were about due for a haircut when we came here. When Jane comes back, I'm going to ask if there's a barber who could come in and give you a trim. Unless you want me to try."

Damion's eyes shot me a "Don't you dare!" look.

"Teasing, D.," I said. "I know the damage I've done with scissors before. I won't ever cut your hair again, I promise. Are you sleepy? Why don't you just drift back to sleep. I'll sit by you quietly, and I won't even think of cutting your hair."

Marnix was still busy talking to Dr. Sastry and Dr. Brodsky out at the center of the unit. He bent over the desk, looking at long strips of echocardiographs from last night. Dr. Brodsky was pointing to them and speaking quietly with him. Dr. Sastry listened, nodding his head rhythmically in between other interruptions like the phones and nurses asking him questions.

Damion was already asleep, worn out from his bath. I got up to slide the glass door nearly closed to block out the unit's daytime clatter of voices from other visitors and carts being wheeled across the shiny floor. Damion slept well in the bright morning light, and I myself was lulled by the repetition of the numbers flashing on his monitor and the exhalation of the ventilator.

The sun streaming in the window had the same happy clarity of the morning light that used to flood into the southern exposure of his windows in our old house. This morning's light made me think of a bedroom I painted for him when he was a toddler. It made me think about a small and beautiful fragment of our past together, just a little scene that made me smile for a minute.

JUNE 1981

When Damion was fourteen months old, with a new brother on the way in a month, Marnix and I talked about moving him out of his nursery. Feeling guilty about this early eviction, I made a promise, "I'm going to paint a brand new bedroom for you, D. I'm going to make it like the inside of a special book, like this one. And you can have a big boy's bed. You'll even be closer to Dadda and Momma's room."

Before the month was out, and far enough in advance of the new baby's arrival that he might not connect the two events, Damion was moved to a room that would have made Lewis Carroll proud. It was a garden of a room, with a wraparound mural lifted out of *Alice in Wonderland*. There were garden walls, topiaries, grass and sky. Above the toy box, The White Rabbit trumpeted, making this a most important looking corner. Alice was on her knees in the grass, surprised. Tweedle Dee and Tweedle Dum were interlocked between the windows, looking very confused and silly. Silly enough for Damion to charge the wall, slap his fat hands on their rotund bellies and squeal out, "Mans!"

And Humpty-Dumpty. How could I not have painted him? He balanced precariously over the bed, grinning confidently, oblivious to the danger. Thinking he was immune. He had no idea of his vulnerability. No idea at all. Just like most of the world still. Just like us back then.

Oh, D., I thought, maybe it was a terrible mistake to paint Humpty-Dumpty there, a terrible omen.

TUESDAY AFTERNOON

At lunch, Marnix caught me up on this morning's medical picture. "Brodsky feels that although the fluid is obviously reaccumulating, last night's echo and today's chest x-rays make him think that it isn't as much as before the two taps. And although there is a mild degree of mitral insufficiency, he wants to wait and see what happens."

"That sounds better than what you felt last night. That's encouraging isn't it, if he wants to watch and wait?"

"Yes. And another encouraging thing is that the lungs are looking more clear on the chest films today. The bad thing is that Damion's heart is enlarging each time they shoot another x-ray. That's bad. Brodsky wants to watch the cardiomegaly like a hawk. Expect a portable chest x-ray every few hours.

"But the lungs look so much better that Dr. Sastry's going to remove the left chest drainage tube later this afternoon."

"That's what we love. Things coming out. This is the first thing to come out, isn't it? Yeah, it is," I answered myself. "I think you should start eating more, dear. You're getting really thin. Here, please eat some of this. I got too much." Most of the time Marnix simply forgot to eat. "So, it sounds like the lungs are clearing and he might get the respirator out tomorrow after all. One tube is going out later today. His heart is holding its own, although it's bad that it continues to enlarge."

Marnix nodded while he chewed on some of my sandwich. He rarely had an appetite these days. I was glad to see he was acting hungry now.

"It's the fluid again, isn't it? That's what's blowing up the image of his heart, isn't it?"

After he swallowed and chased down his food with some of my milk, he explained, "You see how this disease is unfolding. You can see how it behaves. It's one hit after another. It ricochets around from one organ to another. You never can anticipate where the next hit will occur or when it will stop."

"The roller coaster," I said.

"Yes. Apparently Damion's kidneys are starting to improve. His urine output is better and his BUN is coming down. The lungs have taken a beating, but it looks like there's hope there. The heart's the big question mark now. It's obviously getting the next whack."

I asked about what was scaring me the most. "How do you feel about the neurological picture? He's not having any more of those little short circuited lapses of confusion, but I worry about how sleepy and withdrawn he's becoming."

"I don't know. We just have to hope that all that was temporary and that the sleepiness comes from the general beating he's taken. He can throw a clot any time. You know that. But at least we're aggressively going after him with plasmapheresis. I swear that's kept him from a serious infarct or a fatal hit so far."

"Sounds like we're in a holding pattern, maybe a bit of a respite from where we were."

"If we asked what classification he is today, as opposed to some of the rougher days he's been through, what do you think they'd say?"

Marnix thought about it a moment before he answered. "Whereas he was 'critical,' he might now be called in 'stable but serious condition.'"

"That's good, dear. That's much better." I didn't even think of the irony. Any improvement made me grateful.

When we put our tray onto the funny conveyor belt that shuttled them to the kitchen for washing, I thought of one thing I wanted to do before getting back on the elevator. "I'm going to look for some paper or cards to write to the children. Do you want me to get you something from the shop? Or more cash from the ATM machine in the lobby while I'm down there?"

"No, we're still okay. See you up there."

"See you." And we split as the hallways forked.

Another unexpected series of drops in our roller coaster ride. Setbacks with Damion's plasma exchange. Physical ones. Bigger political ones. "Does this mean we have to stop?" I asked Marnix who had just returned from talking with Dr. Cahil outside Damion's room.

Damion's torso and arms were streaked and splotched with angry tentacles of red. The patterns resembled seaweed. They looked like the August in Panama City when all the seaweed had washed in and we let the children wallow in the tepid water. Damion popped up waist deep in it and called to me on the shore, "Look, Mom, I'm a sea monster!" Now, again, he was draped in long strands. This time they were part of him and they were a flaming red.

"John says no. We can't afford to. He's going to talk to Cahil again now on the phone," Marnix answered.

"But I got the strong impression that Dr. Cahil was about to recommend against any more exchanges when he saw this reaction.

Are we doing the right thing? Is it getting more dangerous?"

"Not as dangerous as allowing the hemolysis to rebound. We cannot back off," he answered firmly.

"What's Kelton saying about it? What are the specific points he makes?"

"That if we stop too soon, Damion's going to fall back into a hole that he can't get out of. Did you see this morning's platelet count? 85,000! Sunday's was 55,000. Four days ago they were 38,000, and a day before that they bottomed at 14,000. That's way back up the hill for us. He's pulling out of a nose dive.

"If we stop now, we could slide back to where no amount of plasmapheresis could help once everyone panicked and tried to resume it." Marnix was resolute. I knew he had Dr. Finley at the blood bank supporting him. I had seen the notes Marnix wrote of their initial conversation. I saw the notation that the plan was to exchange Damion's plasma daily and that the goals were a platelet count of at least 125,000, with a stable DH and hemoglobin.

I knew that John Kelton was walking everyone through the process of how much to do and when to do it and the meaning of specific blood factor levels on Damion's frequent hematology lab reports.

I saw one emphatic notation on Marnix's list after he spoke with John on Saturday. It seemed most pertinent now. In huge letters underlined twice, it commanded:

DON'T STOP PHERESIS
EVEN WHEN PLATELETS 100,000!!!!

All of this continued to be of formidable help. But some of the doctors were becoming more and more reluctant, less and less appreciative of Marnix taking such a determined role in this. And now Danny was gone on vacation. If Dr. Sastry sided with Dr. Cahil or Havis on this, we were outvoted. Marnix knew that today's reaction put the continuation of plasmapheresis in peril.

"So Danny's not here now. Who decides? You? Sastry? Cahil?"

Marnix didn't answer my rhetorical question. He distractedly handled one of the IV lines, tapping a tiny trapped bubble along its length of liquid. He was thinking of the dilemma. He was also thinking of a last resort contingency plan of moving Damion, maybe even by air ambulance, if we had to. But a transfer would be messy and risky and perhaps impossible with all the complications and fragility of his condition. Marnix barely breathed his thoughts to me. To talk might invite them into the realm of possibility. But I had found him looking in the Yellow Pages under air ambulance services. And he had hinted to me that we'd move him.

I held Damion's upper arm as he slept on. The streaks frightened me.

WEDNESDAY, MARCH 11
"This is the big day, the appointed day for Damion to get off the respirator."

"It looks encouraging," Marnix agreed. "The final two films last evening and last night looked good, except for his heart, and the radiology reports both indicated the lungs are essentially clear."

"Do you think he'll be able to drink right away?"

"I talked with Kiros about that during his afternoon rounds. Don't expect this to be easy, Mary. It's going to be slow going getting his digestive tract back in working order. Yesterday's abdominal film shows he still has a rough looking colon and a lot of inflammation and gaseous distention in both the large and small bowel. So don't get your hopes up that he can start eating and drinking anytime soon. It's going to be clear liquids for a few days at least."

"That's okay. As long as he can drink a little. All his favorite drinks are clear anyway." I thought of how many times he'd brought up Sprite in the last week.

"All right, let's get in there. I'm going to run ahead. You come when you're ready."

"Be there in one minute."

When I came into Damion's room, I found him surrounded by Marnix, Dr. Sastry and someone from Respiratory Therapy. Damion was red faced and crying silently behind the hoses. When he saw me, he pointed vigorously to the note he'd scrawled onto the board.

"THEY'RE BREAKING THEIR PROMISE!!" it complained pitifully.

"What is it?" I asked the men. "Why aren't you taking him off the respirator?"

The respiratory therapist was shaking his head firmly.

Dr. Sastry distantly argued, "It's not the right thing to do now. Yes, the lungs are looking clear on the recent films, and one chest tube is out. But we've had only one day of clear pictures for his lungs. There is still an area of underaeration at the left medial base. There is still this enlarged heart and it looks like the heart may be compressing the left lower lobe."

The respiratory therapist added for Marnix and me, "I don't see any reason to rule out atelectasis at this point." Then he looked into Damion's eyes and said, "It's too early. It would be premature to take you off it now. You could end up having to struggle if we let you breathe room air on your own, buddy."

I knew he was right. But I also knew that if anything had kept Damion hanging on since the previous Thursday, it was his fixation on the goal that Danny laid out for him. I worried that if we withdrew this hope from him, he would withdraw further into the disease, thinking all deals were off.

Marnix leaned down closer to Damion and said, "Baby, I know how much you counted on this. It hurts us all to have to change our minds. You know that we have to do the best thing for you."

Damion nodded his head as hot tears were wiped away by his father's hands. He lifted the tablet in resignation and wrote, "Now how long do I have to wait?" and held it up for all of us.

"We'll assess as we go along," Dr. Sastry said more to the therapist and Marnix than he did to Damion. "We'll just have to wait and see."

Marnix gave Damion the answer he needed. "We're not going to make any promises we might not be able to keep. Every time we get another chest x-ray or an echo, and every time someone from respiratory comes up to check on you and the machine, this is going to be the one big question we'll all be asking ourselves. The question that's going to be everybody's priority: 'When is the soonest we can get Damion off the breathing tube?' That's what everybody's going to ask."

The therapist patted Damion's foot on tl
as he and Dr. Sastry quietly departed. Dami
toward the wall. We pulled up two chairs to th
his bed. We could see from the profile of his tl
eyes were blinking for ten to fifteen minutes.
steadily onto his hand.

Then he fell asleep.

WEDNESDAY, LATE MORNING

He slept. He slept away the entire day. I sat by him while
Marnix alternated talking to the Blood Bank, gathering up the latest lab reports, checking on what Dr. Havis felt about the last two
days' renal picture, and conferring with Dr. Brodsky when he came
in to compare yesterday's four chest films against this morning's
early portable x-ray. Marnix had a lot to keep up with. He never
dropped in his energy and attention levels to all the facets of
Damion's medical care. He did this without being obstructive or too
intense. I know he was making a big effort to give all the specialists
their space, to assume a calm, methodical approach. However, I
knew inside he was intense.

Marnix came back when he had anything new and substantial to relay. We talked quietly when the nurse stepped out for brief
periods of time. Damion was in a deep enough sleep. The respirator sounds drowned out any chance of us waking him. Most of
today's information was decent news. Most of it was encouraging
from a physical standpoint. Only, I couldn't help being uneasy
about what impact this morning's disappointment would have on
Damion's spirits.

"Dr. Havis went over the trends in his chemistry profiles over
the last two days. BUN is inching down now. Remember the high
was ninety-five Saturday? Well, it's creeping down now to the low
seventies," he said happily.

"Any feeling about the dialysis?" I asked, looking at the three
bags of blood-tinted fluid under his bed. The machine was in its
purge cycle. "I mean, not that we're asking to get our hopes dashed
by looking forward to a specific date for another piece of machinery, but is Dr. Havis giving you any hint of when that will be safe to
discontinue?"

"No, not really. No discussion of that, but peritoneal dialy-sis is working well for Damion."

"So, his kidneys are still battered but they look hopeful? Is that about right?" I felt guilty for feeling hostile about the respira-tor disappointment.

"Yes, he's hanging in there from a nephrologist's point of view."

"Okay. Thanks, Marnix. I guess that is good news. Just like the infiltrate clearing out of his lungs and one chest tube taken out. We don't need everything collapsing at once, do we? And what time do you think the Blood Bank is coming?" I asked, to change the topic to one that I knew energized and gave him hope.

"About two. Let's just hope Dr. Cahil isn't hanging around. Or if he is, that the skin reaction doesn't recur."

WEDNESDAY AFTERNOON

Bags of plasma were lined up on the bed again, the precious gift of many donors in each one. The whining plasma exchange machine infused two more liters of fresh frozen plasma as it simul-taneously drew off the two-liter volume of plasma in Damion's blood.

The skin reaction did not recur. There were no angry streaks, no signs of reaction at all to ruin the afternoon. Only pale skin as the shrill cycling machine churned and churned through its two hours of duty. It sounded like the loud ice cream maker I had at home—its motor made the same pitched noise, only louder.

This was Damion's seventh exchange. The only day he missed was last Thursday when he was too critical because of res-piratory failure and that evening's close call with his blood pressure. But every day other than that darkest day revolved around this ther-apy and its hope.

Dr. Cahil entered the room as the treatment was about half way through. His dark Middle Eastern eyes watched quietly, pen-sively. He didn't project the same alarm and authoritarianism as yesterday. After a few tense moments, he asked for Marnix to step outside the sliding glass door.

Through it I watched Marnix unfold one of his notebook papers he used to scribble lab values on. I knew what he was preparing to say to Dr. Cahil. The steady climb in platelet count was rising in ten to fifteen point increments every time the lab sent up another report to the P.I.C.U. station. By now, the nurses automatically ripped these off the printer and brought them to Marnix, unless Dr. Sastry was at the desk, in which case they showed them to him first. Last night's 6:30 results were the last Marnix had a definitive number on. It was up to ninety-nine, fifteen points higher than yesterday morning's 5:00 A.M. sampling. I knew Marnix's intent was to stand by the numbers, to defend the strategy by showing evidence of its success. Dr. Cahil, of course, was tracking all these numbers too and then some, but Marnix must have felt in their conversation that he had to produce them. It was not a long conversation, not nearly as long as some of the discussions they got into. Dr. Cahil had the advantage of age and specialty. His posture was that of the one in charge. Marnix assumed the body language of a respectful pupil. Then, Dr. Cahil nodded his dignified nod and walked out of the unit. Marnix refolded his paper and returned to Damion, the blood bank nurse, and me.

His eyes flashed a quick notation to me: It's okay.

We resumed our mesmerizing focus on the exchange. The plasma still exited the output tube of Damion's femoral line as thicker and darker than the plasma being infused. Toxins were being removed in this purulent fluid.

Marnix and I felt this was saving his life.

How could we know?

We couldn't.

We just prayed it would.

Someone from the mail room had started to make daily trips to Damion's corner of the unit. People from our hometown heard about his condition on Sunday morning in church and Monday morning in school and sent him an abundance of letters and packages. I poured through them and found the task a welcome distraction from our vigil. There were small packages with books and little toys, at least forty cards, a package from his class with a long computer banner, and letters from each classmate. There were construction paper cards made by all of Mila's classmates in the second grade. An encouraging letter came from Damion's headmaster.

Another inspirational letter came from his school basketball coach. The soccer coach wrote that the boys would all write and promised to pick up medals and T-shirts for him at every tournament until he rejoined them. Uncle Ben and Aunt Susan sent letters and a chocolate dinosaur. Aunt Grace sent a little hand held massager from Sharper Image. The outpouring of love was truly overwhelming. There were even kind and caring letters to Marnix and me, many from people who were only slight acquaintances.

Damion awoke to all the mail and presents which had been sent from home piled up beside him on the bed. I opened the envelopes for him, and he looked at each card and read its contents. The things that meant the most to him, judging by his concentration, were the letters and drawings of his classmates. Most of the boys wrote macho little notes like, "Damion, hope your nurses are babes. Now get out of there soon. We need you in basketball during recess." Two of the boys who were good artists drew fanciful pictures of what they imagined hospital life to be like. The most creative soul of all started a comic strip for Damion of little vignettes that happened at school in Damion's absence. They were fascinating cartoons, recognizable caricatures of kids in the class, a great series that he'd elaborate on in future installments.

"Who is this kid, D.?" I asked. "He's a sheer genius."

The girls wrote sympathetic, sweet notes to him, telling how much they missed him at his desk, and imploring him to get well and come back. Their notes were nearly weepy and loaded with little bits of sentimentality in the form of flowers all over the page. It was obvious that they were upset. I never imagined so many ways a heart could be put into a picture before I looked at their representations. There were pumping hearts, hearts dripping out of the clouds, timid hearts with flowers growing in their boundaries, bursting hearts. "These girls are very sweet. You're so lucky to have a class where the girls and boys are all such good buddies for one another."

Halfway through this largesse, I saw it was time to let him rest. "We'll save some for later. What do you want me to do with all this good stuff! How about if I hang up this banner and the cards you've read?" He pointed to the banner and then to the space high up on the wall he faced. I turned to his nurse Pepper who was listening while rehanging one of his IV bags. "Is that okay if we hang these up? I'll keep them only on the glass door and this wall, away from all the complicated things."

Pepper stretched her body, one hand on the IV pole, the other hand over the plastic basin with dressing supplies. She tossed a roll of surgical tape at me and said, "Do it, girl. Get rid of some of this drab. You can stick some of that on me, too and I'll wear it around for you, Damion. I'll be a walking get-well card."

Damion's eyes narrowed into little slits of a smile before he closed them for sleep. Pepper kept on working and I climbed on a chair to hang up the banner high above the door to a bathroom Damion had never used.

"He's pretty bummed out about the ventilator," she said to me once he was asleep. "I guess he really had it in his mind that today was the day the suffering would end, huh?"

"Yes. He was counting on getting at least one break," I answered and looked over to make sure he'd fallen asleep.

WEDNESDAY EVENING

After dinner on the way back to our room to clean up before we started the night's vigil, Marnix and I heard voices from the formerly unoccupied parents' room across the hall. It sounded like many people inside. There were lots of voices of several people talking at once. As we were going into our room, their door opened. Inside, the room was packed with bags, blankets, pillows, and seven or eight adults. A dark-haired man in his twenties in creased gray sweats was coming out.

"Hello," I said.

He looked stunned. And as the door widened all the people in the room had become silent, and they all looked stunned. Some had red eyes as if they had been crying. Their focus shifted to Marnix and me pushing on our door. The young man answered awkwardly with a flat, "Hi" and kept walking head down to the P.I.C.U. doors that were opposite our set.

"Uh oh," I said to Marnix when we got inside our room. "Someone else is in trouble."

13

The Spectre

I SAW THE DARK-HAIRED young man again while I sat alone eating breakfast. The stranger was sitting with a piquant faced young woman at the next table. As they drank their coffee, I noticed that they wore matching wedding bands. When I finished my plate of grits and eggs, I got up to put my tray away and paused at their table.

"Hi. I'm across the hall from you in the other room for parents of children in intensive care. If there's anything my husband and I can do, knock on our door."

As I said it, I realized this was a meaningless offer. What could we possibly do for this family, we who were numbed by our own pain and Damion's illness? The husband brightened, but his wife continued to stare ahead, her lip trembling but otherwise expressionless.

"What are y'all in for?" he asked as if we were serving prison terms.

"Our eleven-year-old has a disease called H.U.S. A blood and kidney disorder. It's pretty bad. He's had lots of complications."

The man nodded. "Our little boy is up there, too. He had his second birthday less than a month ago."

His wife began to cry.

"Listen," I said, "They're very good here. The doctors and nurses are outstanding."

The man seemed to need to talk about what happened. "He fell into our swimming pool. He wasn't out of sight for more than a minute. My wife looked out the window and saw him floating."

I felt the black hole of guilt surrounding this little boy's mother. I knew it would never release her from its force.

"He's gonna come back. He's gonn[a]
father said with conviction to me and an imp[...]
mother stopped crying and stared blankly thro[ugh]
scenes whirling around her.

After fumbling for a way to comfort them, I starte[d]
to the unit. He called after me, "Hey! You wanna know hi[s]
name? Boo Man. He's always darting off and finding places to h[ide.]
When he pops out, he shouts, 'Boo!' What's yours named?"

"Damion. We call him 'D.' Or sometimes 'Animal.'"

"We'll see ya around while Boo Man and D. get better.
Right?"

"Right!" I said, smiling at him.

I looked at his grieving wife. She was gone, pulled into a
black space that her husband couldn't see.

THURSDAY AFTERNOON

While we sat through the afternoon's plasma exchange, I
mulled over the rapid weight loss I saw in Damion that had become
more pronounced as the days went on. I saw it with greater clarity
this day as the sun bathed his face in a light that heightened his
angularity. His boniness horrified me. A whiteness and a skeletal
thinness cried at me, "Look. This is the spectre of your child's
death. This is the look of death approaching." I had never thought
about how my children's skulls might look under their round and
precious faces. Who would? Now, the thought intruded like an evil
presence that came to sit beside us.

There was a scale mechanism built into the bed and they
tracked Damion's weight every day.

"Terri, how much has he lost?" I asked, frightened to learn
the answer but unable to quell my words.

"Seventeen pounds."

"Seventeen pounds," I repeated looking at Marnix.

My heart pounded fearfully.

"This TPN, Marnix. Can't we crank it up? Can't Damion get
more calories and protein? He's starving even with it."

"Mary," he said quietly. "They're continuing to moderate
this every day according to the blood work. There's only so much
his liver can handle. You can only infuse what the body can accept."

1 get actual digestion going or
time. This has got to be robbing
ghting."

eld up his hand in a gesture of frustra-
ression that everything possible was being
but I was losing my own faith.

NG

x, listen to this. These articles on H.U.S. mention a
er called zero-one-five-sev—"

ust a minute, Mary. John's coming to the phone."

"Sorry."

Lying on his bed, I waited for Marnix to finish his call. I continued reading to myself from the thick manila envelope with medical articles that had come today from my brother-in-law, a dark and humorous angel of Lebanese descent, who was a pediatric ophthalmologist trained by my dad. We owed a lot to Paul. In fact, he introduced Marnix and me. I looked at the thick stack of material he'd dug up. The cover sheet was stamped "National Interactive Retrieval Services."

The packet contained a wealth of information. One article in particular caught my eye: It said that the incidence of H.U.S. was increasing dramatically.

As I waded through the articles, I found that recurring number, 0157:H7. It was the name of a pathogenic strain in the E. coli family that was consistently associated with H.U.S. The article told how the bacteria attach to and ulcerate the intestinal mucous lining. It described how toxins produced by E. coli 0157:H7 are "cytotoxins."

"What's this word mean?" I wrote on a pad and carried it to Marnix. "*CYTOTOXIN????*"

He scribbled the answer without pausing in his conversation. "Kills cells."

I began reading again. There was a section on how these cell-killing toxins break through the endothelial layer of the intestine and spill out into the bloodstream setting up a domino effect of microangiopathic injury.

I walked back with another question. "*Microangiopathic?*"

Marnix wrote, "Damages small blood vessels."

"It's all mapped out," I said to myself. Someone had done the work on the pathology of how Damion's disease unfolded. I skipped down and found that number again. It was everywhere in these papers.

I came upon another article on the diseases H.U.S. and T.T.P. and saw the same searing word my father repeatedly asked me: etiology. Under it was a passage that branded me with its defining heat. "The epidemiological data strongly support that O-one-five-seven:H-seven is the most likely cause of H.U.S., perhaps accounting for up to ninety-five percent of all cases."

"This is it. I found it," I whispered to myself. I was almost overcome. "This is it."

But then, as if finding etiology was not enough, I read another article in the British medical journal *Lancet*. "One to four percent of American retail samples of red meat . . ."

My God, I thought, would this become an epidemic? How many adults and children would be infected?

Now I was scorched with anger and sick to my stomach.

"It's all here. It's all completely and nauseatingly here . . ."

The tightness that had gripped my throat since Damion got sick now radiated down to my stomach and gave me the irresistible urge to throw up. I hurried into the bathroom, lifted the seat, and knelt beside the commode. Nothing came up. I felt only rolling waves of realization that all of this was known, that this detective work on how Damion got sick was well advanced within an elite segment of the medical community, that the implicated bacteria 0157:H7 was responsible for "the dramatic increase" of this disease, that the animal host was identified, and that the vehicle of infection was fecally contaminated meat.

I looked down at the paper again. Incredulous. Meat. Meat could kill. Meat was what infected Damion. If he died, it would be because of contaminated meat. Something tainted fed to him by people there to protect him. It was too much to absorb.

Marnix finished his conversation and came through the cracked bathroom door. I had given up trying to vomit; I feared this was a nausea that I was going to have to stomach, the sickening burden of knowing too much.

"What's the matter, Mary?"

"John's right. It *was* meat. It's really sickening to find out about something evil the hard way with no warning at all. Have you heard anything about a virulent new bacteria in our meat supply? Have you ever heard anything about needing to cook meat until it's well done? Nobody knows about this. Nobody's warning people. We got no warning at all for Damion. Nothing. How many people will die because they don't know?"

Marnix pulled me off the floor. He was overcome with sadness. He said, "I'm not going to read those. I can't now. My focus is going to be on how Damion can bail out of this disaster, okay? You read all of it. You go ahead and learn what you can. I have to give my attention to walking Damion through this minefield. Do you understand?"

I nodded. "Yes. I don't know if I can stomach all this now, either. The kind of issues this material raises are so ominous that I'm unsure that I can even think about them now. Maybe I have to put this stuff away in the envelope and concentrate on it later." I turned to him. "Marnix, there's one mention that antibiotics and antidiarrheal drugs can lead to higher morbidity for H.U.S. Do you know how much Pepto-Bismol and Emetrol I forced Damion to take on that Saturday and Sunday? I probably made this worse. I could be the one factor that tipped him into H.U.S. You don't know how sorry I am if I did."

"You can't feel bad about that," Marnix said as he firmly gathered up all the articles and placed them back in the envelope. "A significant number of doctors would treat every case with Damion's symptoms just as you did, throw antibiotics at him. It's the 'fix-it' American way," he said.

"Ignorance is bliss, isn't it, Marnix?"

"It's usually blissful, but sometimes deadly."

Marnix put the envelope of articles in the dresser drawer and slid it under all the pads we had used so far to track Damion's lab work and reports.

"Let's get something to eat." He held out his big hand to me and I clasped it gratefully, but the revolting information I'd read was locked in me forever.

THURSDAY NIGHT

I was alone in the unit with Damion. Marnix couldn't stay awake much past ten; so I told him I'd wait up and see who the nurse was on the eleven o'clock shift. I was racked by my guilt and knew it would be impossible for me to go to sleep until I was very tired. At least there by Damion I could watch him. A bright fluorescent light seeped into his cubicle from the central desk area where all the nurses congregated. At least there was no deafening quiet as in our room. The respirator sounds had provided a hypnotic background music for Damion's disease for eight straight days now. It was a backdrop of endless regularity, the airy inhalation and deflating exhalation. I thought of how the eight days on the respirator must feel from his perspective. For Damion I knew it was not only a mechanical forcing of air into his chest. It was a sound that whispered enslavement and a lack of freedom to breathe as his body and mind instructed him. He had no choice. The machine's tempo dictated the timing of each breath. In submitting physically to the ventilator, he had to surrender something of himself. I was sure of this tonight. I was sure that I'd arrived at one of the explanations of how this strong and positive child had been reduced to a depressed and withdrawn patient. He had to submit his body and its rhythms to the tyranny of a machine.

Damion knew intellectually that the respirator was something he needed. But physically he had to experience it as something that denied him drinking. Worse, he'd learned that the respirator was something that periodically betrayed him. Once every few hours, the hoses had to be unplugged from the machine and drained of all the moisture that condensed in them. "Hang on, Damion," his nurse would shout at him. "The air's coming back on in a minute. Just hold your breath while I pour this water out. Hang on just a second, honey."

Sometimes the fluid backed up in the tube that ran down his throat and occluded the air opening. There was no way he could anticipate this mishap, and, when it happened, it happened quickly. We'd see him gag and choke, reach for the nurse's arm, and then be helpless waiting for someone to rescue him. All the unit nurses knew about this eventuality and came immediately to detach the hose from the tube and suction out his plastic airway.

So the respirator represented thirst, discomfort, and danger to him, even though he understood our explanation of how it allowed his battered lungs to function. The respirator was a perfect metaphor for the whole disease, as far as I was concerned. There were no clear-cut answers, no easy way out, and no uncomplicated way to stop the roller coaster's course. Everything became a trade-off or a choice clouded with contradictions and drawbacks.

These were the sleepy thoughts that inhaled and exhaled in and out of me as the night passed. Life was becoming one continuum of bad news.

Suddenly the wooden doors flew open. In strutted M.T., the shapely brunette nurse everyone eyed. She was an effervescent powerhouse of a person in her early twenties. Apparently her humor was legendary on the pediatrics floor. I had only seen her once before late one night when we'd first come. At that time she shocked me with her immodest and loud jokes with the other nurses. Tonight M.T. burst into the unit with an astonished toddler in her arms. The little girl in a cartoon patterned hospital gown looked too amazed to move, yet somehow she seemed secure and happy in M.T.'s grasp.

"STUDLY!" M.T. hollered in our direction. "Hey! What'd you do with my stud?" she demanded of the nurses at the desk. "What'd you do? Move him on me?"

One of the nurses shook her head in amusement and pointed to the other side of the unit. "He's in there."

M.T. marched over to baby Marty's door. "Stud! Wake up, Studly Marty! I found you a woman!"

The little girl gnawed on her fist as M.T. stood over baby Marty's crib. A smiling Saracita walked in to pull Marty upright against the metal bars. He wobbled as he held on tight, his face sleepy but full of fascination. He opened his mouth in the way that babies do to squeal in happy surprise.

"Check her out, Marty! Isn't she hot? She's a pretty little girl, isn't she? Marty, you know that I'm always lookin' out for you."

I watched Marty's fat legs pumping up and down with delight.

"Here, y' all hold hands now for a minute. This is your first date." M.T. held onto the little girl who fingered Marty's face and gingerly examined the hose that plugged into his neck. Saracita steadied Marty's back as he stood erect and serious when the baby girl touched his face.

"Okay, kids. I better get back to work. You know I love my fat Marty, but M.T.'s got to go now. But I'll be bringing you other women, whenever I find them out there on the floor for you."

After a few moments she uncurled the baby girl's hands from Marty's. Then M.T. said softly to her, "Say bye bye to Marty. Wave bye bye. Say nighty night, little Mr. Potato Head."

Marty stood still as M.T. and the baby backed away. "See, Marty, she loves you! I told you you're a natural stud."

FRIDAY, MARCH 13

"Friday the thirteenth," I said half ominously to myself in the mirror. I was brushing my teeth after breakfast. Marnix was still in Damion's room talking to the doctors who drifted in and out on their morning rounds. I'd never considered before that superstitions deserved any kind of acknowledgment. But lately there were a lot of things I never previously considered that now rudely imposed themselves on my belief system.

"What kind of further bad things can happen today?" I wondered as I started to brush my bottom teeth. In the mirror, I took note of my appearance. "You are looking bad, Mary," I told myself, dispassionately. My skin looked as though I hadn't been outside in weeks, which was true. And dark roots showed where I lightened my bangs. My whole image looked rather hopeless to me; so I found a hairclip on the glass shelf under the mirror and pulled back my hair, threw on some lipstick and blush to counter the wan look, and left it at that.

Marnix came into our bedroom, grabbed hold of me and held me tight. "Congratulations, Mary. Oh, congratulations!"

This was not what I had envisioned a moment ago when I thought of the looming misfortune of Friday the thirteenth.

"Platelets are up to normal range. He's climbing out of the hole!" Marnix rocked me in a celebratory hug. Then he reached in his pants pocket and produced the lab report. "Here, I'll show you. This is from a sample collected at six-o-five this morning. A vigorous thirty-four thousand-point jump from last night's. Look, it's the first reading we've seen without an 'L' for low, beside it. This is good. It's very good. A hundred and fifty-eight thousand! God, I'm so happy. John's going to be so glad when he hears this. Damion's crawling out of it. Plasma exchange is pulling him out of it."

"This means we can stop now?" I asked hopefully.

"No. Not yet."

"Didn't Dr. Finley say the usual blood bank goals are to continue until a hundred and twenty-five thousand? I thought that was our goal."

"John's been talking with me about it over the last couple of days as it looked like we were going to cross this line. He tells me that's a common big mistake. Second only to beginning too late is stopping too soon. Yes, the platelets are at the low end of normal range now. But there are other considerations hematologically speaking. Damion could still slide back at this stage. However, we are entering a new phase. And that's what's so beautiful to me."

Marnix assumed a more ominous tone before continuing.

"All right. We are curing the underlying disease, but we are vulnerable to complications. 'Cure the disease and the complications can kill you,'" he quoted solemnly.

"That's just great. How reassuring," I said sarcastically. I knew there had to be overtones of Friday the Thirteenth in there somewhere. "So, the roller coaster's out of the nosedive, but Damion can still crash and burn. You mean that he still can die. He's getting beyond the underlying disease process, but he still can die."

"Mary, you know that's a given with his condition. We can't think about that today. We have to be grateful that he's gotten to this. We've got to be grateful. Please remember that."

"Okay." I put my head under his arm. When we hug, I come up to the height of his armpit, so I get this wonderful feeling of being enfolded. "Okay, Marnix, I'm really happy the platelets are up. I'm really happy that we are on the threshold of a new level for Damion. The beast is beaten back. So now, the focus is just not to let its damage kill him."

Marnix told me the plan. "We're going to plasmapherese until we get every assurance that any mopping up it can accomplish is done. Until John says 'enough.' And we're going to mop up the damage the disease has done to each organ, one by one. There's still a lot of danger. But the disease is unraveling now."

"Congratulations, Marnix, dear."

"Congratulations, Mary."

We held each other a moment more. Then we stood apart.

He said, "Okay, come with me. Dr. Sastry called Dr. Brodsky to do another echo. The x-ray showed more collapsed lung tissue. And it showed heart enlargement again. He'll be here any time now."

For Marnix's sake I didn't say it, but if the second part of our ambivalent new motto had to do with complications, it sure didn't take long for them to mount their assaults.

This time, Dr. Brodsky performed the echocardiogram himself. Again, he invited Marnix and me to sit and watch. Dr. Brodsky, though still somewhat reserved and understated, was expressing more of his growing impatience. He had tried twice to stop the pericardial effusion that threatened to damage Damion's heart function. Twice he had gone in and drawn off the fluid, leaving behind a tiny surgical drain. And twice the drain had been dislodged and the heart lining continued to produce an amazing volume of fluid, reinflating the ballooning heart silhouette on the screen.

Dr. Brodsky didn't betray what conclusion his frustration led him to, but, as I watched his frowning face reading the patterns and images on the echo, I wondered if he could possibly be thinking the same thing I was. *If these images mean a third tap, Dr. Brodsky, could this be it for Damion?*

Marnix waited until he was ready to explain his findings. Damion lay perfectly still, watching the undulating images of his heart on the angled machine parked against his bed. A child of the computer age, he was less impressed than I was that an image could be transferred by sonar technology from his chest interior into the machine and there be reassembled into a picture of his living, beating heart.

Dr. Brodsky straightened up, ready to give his opinion.

"Okay. I've gotten several views here showing evidence of a significant increase of pericardial effusion. I'd say it looks like it's the same amount as the study three days ago."

I saw Marnix's anxiety flare instantly. He listened for the second part of the report.

Dr. Brodsky motioned for us to come closer to the screen. "See this?"

Marnix said, "I think so, yes. The right ventricle. . . ."

"Correct. Diastolic collapse of the right ventricle."

Marnix nodded at the screen. During these technical exchanges Marnix assumed the part of doctor, not parent. I thought about the blond echocardiography technician who had frustrated Marnix by not sharing results. Thank goodness these doctors didn't do that. Dr. Brodsky's inclusion of Marnix made me like and respect him even more.

I watched the two men bent over the machine. "And see this? Do you see respiratory variation? I think it's indicative of an early form of pulsus paradoxicus. There is some thickening there."

Sidney Brodsky switched the equipment off and pushed back his chair. He looked at Damion. "Anything you want to know?" he asked him.

Damion nodded and reached for his pad and pencil. "*Can you give me something to make it not hurt as much?*"

Dr. Brodsky placed his hand on Damion's shoulder. "That's fair enough, Damion. We'll try our best to keep you from waking up this time."

Marnix and I left the unit and went to the cafeteria. Marnix became Damion's dad once more.

"Marnix, we've done it before. That means we can do it again," I said. I knew my logic was debatable, but I wanted to find some bright side to this, some kind of solace. Marnix didn't even answer.

"Sastry did the right thing calling him in this morning, right?" I knew this was no kind of encouragement either. It was unrelated to the fact that Damion was upstairs right then with a needle through his ribs. But this one sounded reassuring, also.

"Yes, the absolutely right thing. Sastry's been right about this," he agreed, trying also to extract consolation from this peripheral thought.

I was glad we'd come down here for this tap.

"Another good thing is that Dr. Brodsky's had a lot of experience doing this procedure on Damion by now." I could tell from Marnix's expression this was my worst attempt yet to make him feel better, the most clumsy try of all. But he just nodded and said, "Yeah."

Rather than make matters any worse, I hushed and waited out the thirty minutes in silence. Trying to make this better for Marnix and myself was futile. It was better to just sit it out until it passed.

The tap results were the same. Dr. Brodsky reported once again the same reaccumulation of the same serous fluid, the same implantation of a small drain tube on the pericardium. Damion slept more soundly because Dr. Brodsky had honored his request and added more painkiller on top of the local anesthesia. We weren't getting better at handling these taps, but, after Dr. Brodsky left, an air of routine settled around Damion sleeping off the sedative.

FRIDAY AFTERNOON

A new fear began to solidify today. Watching Damion, I saw a dullness about him, a flaccid resigned mentality. His earlier disorientation and irrationality had disappeared after dialysis pulled the poisons out of his bloodstream. The possibility of neurological involvement raised then had subsided. It wasn't only that Damion slept around the clock with brief thirty to forty-five minute waking periods. It was that, when he was awake, he was almost irretrievably distant from us.

Dr. Gunderman continued to watch him closely but he was unable to assess much beyond the gross physical manifestations. Except for the unsedated sleep that overpowered him, these seemed in line. The respirator kept Damion nonverbal; thus, it was hard to get an indication of neurological injury. However, as I thought back I realized there had been plenty of signs. I reviewed the possible transient ischemic attacks, the respiratory failure, and the convulsions when he had his brush with death last Thursday evening. I thought about the edema building up in several of his organs now. What was to prevent his brain from swelling? Stroke, infarct, and ischemia were all possible and common complications.

So, while Damion slept after his tap, I couldn't help but dwell on what he had to lose, maybe what he had already lost. I thought of the conversations Marnix and I had delighted in and expounded upon since Damion as a baby began talking to us.

"God, I'm so glad he has a good brain," Marnix had repeated to me numerous times.

"He is so darned smart," we'd say, nearly giddy over what we had produced.

Was it my father's brilliance? My mother's fast-as-lightning thinking? Opa, too, was respected for his innate intelligence though war in Europe prevented him from getting a higher education. He had risen about as high as you can in life with sheer will and instinct and had used his brain to gain success. This little boy's intelligence came from them. It was a rare gift that made us grateful and allowed us to brag to one another at night.

Was it still intact? Had it been stripped away by some new bacteria called 0157:H7? Did those medical literature references to learning disabilities predict our own fate? *Oh, D.D., please hold tight to your gift. All these people can hang onto your lungs for you. They can fight for your heart and kidneys and your colon. But you have to hold fast to your mind. Is that what you're doing far away from us in your sleep?*

FRIDAY EVENING

Dr. Sastry popped his head into Damion's doorway to check on him.

"What's the scoop?" he asked in an upbeat, booming tone.

Damion hadn't seen him approaching. At the sound of Dr. Sastry's exuberant voice, he startled.

"What's the scoop, Damion?"

Damion tried to motion something with his hands, but neither I nor Dr. Sastry could make sense of what he meant.

"Well, it looks like things are going better," Dr. Sastry said noting the monitor numbers overhead. As he turned to leave, I asked him, "Dr. Sastry, will you be in tomorrow?"

Somehow the thought of the unit slowing down on the weekend didn't occur to me last Saturday when Damion had his second tap and the P.I.C.U. seemed to operate at full tilt. Things just felt quieter here now, and although that could be read as a good sign, I felt concerned about the lull.

"Yes, I'll be in to check."

"Thank you, Dr. Sastry. Good night. And thank you for the help today. We're really glad that's behind him."

Dr. Sastry nodded his head in his very distinctive way. And then he was gone.

SATURDAY, MARCH 14

On Saturday morning, Marnix and I awoke to a plan that seemed to have spontaneously combusted from out of nowhere.

"We'll remove the ventilator today and see how he does on his own," Dr. Sastry told us when he came to the unit in midmorning.

"Oh! Okay. And the chest films? Then the report from radiology looks better?" This was very good news once we realized that it was really here. I felt we had no reason to question its justification. It was only that no one divined any indication of improvement over the last days in Damion's pulmonary edema, or his heart-lung situation in general. At least no one had voiced this plan to us.

"Yes. Here's last night's film and report." He showed it to Marnix, not in the least bit defensively.

I read it with Marnix: "Comparison is made with the study earlier on this day. Left lower lobe infiltrate and atelectasis are present, but the heart size appears to be decreasing slightly. Right lung remains fairly clear."

"Well, yes, this is very good news. How do you go about it?"

"Respiratory Services is on the way up. We'll reduce the mix over a few hours, then if he does well each step of the way, Damion will be extubated and we'll monitor how he does on room air. To wean him off, he may initially require some oxygen. But we'll progressively lower that as he adjusts."

And so, anticlimactically, Damion was finally released from the respirator. Over a period of several hours, the people from respiratory therapy, or R.T. as we'd come to call them, turned down the saturation of oxygen going into his lungs and watched how his blood oxygen saturation numbers responded. The white number informed by the E.T. light on his finger became the focus of the morning. And after everyone's confidence was raised Marnix and I left Damion when the tube was to be removed from his trachea.

In a few minutes, the phone rang in our room. It was one of the nurses at the P.I.C.U. desk.

"Can you send Damion's dad in here? Damion wants to speak with him."

"Yeah, sure. Is everything all right?"

"He's doing fine. But he insists on talking to your husband."

"Do you know about what?"

"No, he just says he has something to tell his father."

"Oh. Sure. Okay. He'll be right there."

I stayed behind since he'd asked specifically to see Marnix. Then, hoping that twenty minutes was enough time for them to be alone together, I went in to see our son myself.

"D.D., welcome back to the world of the talking. You look so good! Say something to me."

"Hi," a scratchy whisper said in response.

"Let me give you a congratulatory kiss. It's so good to hear you again." His face was released from the ghoulish position it had been in for ten days. The surgical tape that contorted his mouth and locked the tube in place was cut and peeled away.

His teeth had been brushed, his mouth washed by long swabs dipped in mouthwash and rubbed over his tongue and gums.

Outside the sliding door, I noticed the power plugs neatly wound and the respirator cart ready to be wheeled back downstairs. The machine and its noise were gone. Damion was free. He was untied from the machine.

I had anticipated that I would be elated seeing him. I wasn't. Instead I felt a wariness. Marnix and I had expected him to be thrilled. He wasn't. He was only subdued, but contented when I pulled a chair up to Marnix and him. I had expected him to finally drink gallons of cold fluids. He didn't. He chewed slowly on a few ice chips. Then he drifted away.

"What did he have to say to you?" I asked Marnix when we knew Damion was asleep. Marnix gestured for me to follow him out of the room. We walked to our room where each of us stretched out on our beds, propping up on our elbows to talk.

"It's amazing. Very impressive what he had to say. Incredible, actually."

"Shoot."

"Well, before I tell you what he told me, let me tell you I was just as impressed by how he told me."

"What do you mean?"

"It was his alertness. His intensity. You know how he's been gone from us a long time now? Sleeping or sleepy? Very foggy, not really here at all?"

"Yes, distant."

"But when he spoke to me just now, there was a clarity I haven't seen in weeks. He was back. Very definite, very earnest, very clear on what he was telling me. Absolutely clear. That's why I believe him."

"What was it?"

"First he said, 'I know what made me sick, Dad.' Then, he told me the dream that he's been having."

As Marnix spoke, I could hear Damion describing what he'd dreamed. I heard it in his own words whispered to his father. I felt the dampness of the campsite, looked up at the overcast slices of sky through the pines. I felt the rumble of hunger in his stomach. In my mind I listened to the other boys' voices, boasting and teasing in their outdoor kitchen as they tried to do what they'd seen their mothers do. Damion had told Marnix:

> It was my job to form the meat into patties. But first I needed to find a way to cut open the big red tube of hamburger meat. I tried a fork. But the plastic wrapper wouldn't rip. Puncturing it did nothing; Mitch Foster was standing around doing something else for dinner. He let me borrow his Scout pocket knife. I sliced right under the words, I.B.P., Dakota City, Nebraska. I wondered what I.B.P. might mean.
>
> "Hey, guys, look what's for dinner. It says so, right on the label: I.B.P. What's that stand for?"
>
> "Intestinal Buffalo Parts," one of the boys cracked.
>
> "Illegal bull pollution," someone else said.
>
> "No, here it is in fine print," I joked. "Incriminating Beef Poop."
>
> "Shut up, Damion."
>
> "You shut up," I teased back.
>
> Mitch's knife sliced easily through the seam and I scooped out

a handful of cool and mushy meat. The core of the meat was bright red, but it had turned grayish brown where it was closer to the edges.

"Hey, does anybody know why meat turns gray like this?"

"Oxygenation. Oxidation. Something like that," someone told me.

"Cool."

It squished in my hands and made wet sticking noises when I pressed it into balls to flatten out for the grill. It was gross. No wonder mothers do all the nasty stuff ahead of time and dads just cook them when they're ready.

Now we were ready and I gave them to someone else who was supposed to put them on the fire. I walked down the path to the creek so I could wash my hands.

Soon we were lining up with white paper plates. The hamburgers were stacked on the tin foil tray I made. I saw one corner that must have gotten knocked off when the burgers were being moved around on the grill. I was starving so I grabbed a little grayish brown piece and popped it in my mouth. But it felt raw and squishy when I chewed it. It must have been like the meat on the outside of the tube: gray from the air. It must not ever have made it to the camp fire like all the other meat. I checked. The other meat was brown all the way through and had burned lines from the grill.

It tasted gross but I didn't want to spit it out in front of my friends. So I just swallowed. Anyway, it wasn't like pork or something that can give you worms if it's not cooked. So I didn't think it could hurt me.

But it did hurt me, didn't it? I have dreamed it over and over again. Each time more parts of it come back to me of how it happened. That's how I know it's what made me sick.

We had never discussed with Damion what was responsible for his illness. He'd never heard "meat" or "food poisoning" mentioned since this whole thing began. "E. coli poisoning" was a term of the future. The only things that shone any light on the dark mystery of etiology were John Kelton's resounding question and the Fed-Ex envelope in our dresser drawer.

Damion arrived at his discovery through another route: a more intuitive, independent, instinctive road that was just as valid. The dreams he had in the last two weeks were long forays into the wilderness. They directed him to the cause of his illness. To me, his journey had great credibility because it was undertaken by the victim, a child who edged along the precipice of death, lingered on its borders, and ventured to a plateau of truth that science could not reach. His dreams had shown him the way to the answer.

SATURDAY LATE AFTERNOON

"Look how dark it's getting out there, Damion. It's about to pour."

The sky outside was leaden now that the afternoon heat had kicked up towering thunderclouds. In a few minutes, they opened up and rain began to pour on Tampa spread out below us. Damion turned his head but he couldn't crane his neck around far enough to see the storm behind his bed. I considered wheeling his bed at an angle but there was no way to move all the associated poles and lines.

"There, look into the mirror on the wall ahead of you. You can see how black the clouds are."

I bent down to Damion's level and checked the angle to be sure he could see. Then I stood to the side of the window to look down on the traffic. The cars had all turned on their headlights and were moving cautiously. Everything slowed down under the violent spring rain, the kind of heavy rain I rarely saw growing up in the North. Here in the South, when clouds unloaded the Gulf's moisture they dumped down a powerful rain that turned streets into small rivers. Now it was pouring over Martin Luther King Boulevard. The hamburger place across the street looked empty and sullen, despite its garish neon. No one was going in or out of the surrounding clinics or the bank.

Even though I was on the top floor and enveloped in the swirling clouds that swept around the building, the storm felt distant. The consequences of water slapping the ground and its impact on human activities like traffic and business seemed remote. The thunder outside that would make children cover their ears and gasp was muffled to a low rumble. Reduced to a growl, it vibrated against my hand on the double window panes. The lightning that would feel snappingly dangerous if I was down there on that sidewalk seemed a special effect, a theatrical flashing over the backdrop of a city under siege.

The hospital was hermetically sealed from the weather, from the outside world for that matter. The hospital was a tight, slightly suffocating, vacuum-sealed shell that was keeping my son alive. He was still alive. He was still alive. The words struck a rainlike cadence in my brain. *It's raining like hell out there, and He's still alive in here.*

SATURDAY EVENING

This evening's chest x-ray didn't look so different to me from the more than two dozen I'd seen up to this point. But Dr. Sastry and Marnix pointed out the swollen contours of the heart and studied the amount of powdery fluff in the lungs with great intensity. They read and reread the report written in the mysterious department downstairs and which Marnix translated for me. "Heart's enlarged obviously. The left lung base has subsegmental pockets of collapsed tissue, and the markings on his lungs are more defined. This might be from him having to work harder at breathing away from the respirator, or he could be developing vascular congestion, which means increased fluid inside the blood vessels."

Neither of us commented but we both realized it was not a good report.

Then Marnix and I ran into a pediatric cardiologist on our way back upstairs from dinner. The doctor approached us in a corridor on the ground floor. "Pardon me," he said in a French Canadian accent. "Are you Dr. and Mrs. Heersink?" He touched Marnix's elbow. "I'm Renato Dubois, an associate of Dr. Brodsky."

Dr. Dubois was a tall, refined, prematurely white-haired man. He spoke in a soft and thoughtful way. "I've just done an echocardiogram on your son to follow up on the pericardiocentesis he had yesterday. May I please speak with you about it?"

We found quiet seats between the cafeteria and the lobby. Dr. Dubois told us that the small catheter left on the pericardial sac in hopes of draining it further had fallen out like the others before it. He had seen the chest x-ray and believed the increase in heart size suggested the reaccumulation of the pericardial fluid. Pulmonary edema also showed up on the echo.

"The echo showed a thick pericardial density. To my eye, it has the consistency of a thrombus; I could not see any fluid or strands. The good part is that cardiac function does not appear to be compromised. I could find no evidence of dysfunction, nor evidence of cardiac tamponade at this time."

Nodding, we said nothing.

"I'll be available all weekend if you need me," he said as he departed.

Marnix and I began to make our way through the labyrinthine hallways to the elevator.

"He was nice to come down to find us, wasn't he?"

"Yes," Marnix answered.

"Thrombus. That means a blood clot," I said quietly.

He looked into my eyes. "Yes."

The bell dinged, the lighted arrow turned off, and the doors swung open. We stepped into the elevator packed with visitors and flowers and went up.

SUNDAY MORNING, MARCH 15

"Danny's here!"

"He's back from vacation? But wasn't it supposed to be after the weekend? Thank goodness. Do you think it's just for a few minutes to check on his patients, and that he'll start tomorrow?"

Marnix was on his way out the door. In fact, he never came through it, only popping his head in our room to let me know the good news as I was waking up. I felt guilty for sleeping later than he, but I knew I'd cover for him later that day and that all of this erratic business of sleeping and waking had some underlying logic holding it together somehow.

Rushing into the unit, I found Dr. Plasencia standing by Damion's bedside. My first inclination was to hug him and thank him for coming back. But Danny was radiating something I'd never seen before from him. Something that felt very much like anger filled the room. He stood up abruptly, said hello to me, and left the room.

"What's that about, Marnix? Did he tell you what's wrong?"

Damion was sleeping soundly through the scene—fortunately, I thought. Marnix motioned for me to wait. I could see his eyes watching the desk area and Danny lifting the phone.

"Ah, yes, this is Dr. Plasencia. For my patient, Damion Heersink in P.I.C.U., let me talk to someone about his TPN please."

The nurse came in and slid the door behind her, blocking off any further chance of hearing the details. She busied herself with

the dialysis equipment and made notations on her pad. Then she
left us alone, sliding the door behind her again. Danny was still on
the phone, going through papers and running his fingers along
reports as he continued talking. To get up now and slide the door
open would make it obvious we were eavesdropping.

"What is it? He looks absolutely furious."

"He's angry. He was very surprised to see how much weight
Damion has lost. He told me he was alarmed about his severe calorie and protein *malnutrition*."

"He used that word? Malnutrition?"

Marnix nodded yes, watching while Danny walked back
toward our door. Danny entered and said, "Okay, okay. I've ordered
a reevaluation of his TPN. We'll be increasing the albumin. For all
these other challenges from his heart and lungs, he needs to maintain his resources."

I remembered what Marnix had once told me about what
happens during starvation: the body begins to rob protein where it
can find it. It begins to steal from the muscles and pilfer protein
from the heart. My own heart beat faster.

"When Dr. Havis arrives, I'd like to discuss discontinuation of
peritoneal dialysis. The BUN and Creatinine are still abnormally
high but they're steadily coming down. The urine output is normal
now, so we may be safe in getting him off. Of course, the catheter will
stay in place until we're sure he manages well without it."

I knew Marnix agreed with this kind of approach whole-
heartedly. I had heard him say repeatedly in other situations: get
patients on whatever kind of intervention they need, but get them
off again as soon as possible. He would be as eager as Danny to see
lines and systems coming out.

"How do you think Damion's doing off the ventilator?"

"Well, his oxygen saturation dropped since he's been on his
own. On the other hand, this morning's chest film looks clearer
than last night's. I'm concerned about the atelectasis and infiltrate,
but I think he's doing pretty well breathing on his own. There's
always a danger of becoming reliant on the ventilator. We have to
watch his blood gases and the effort of his respiration very carefully. You'll be seeing Respiratory Therapy up here as often as when he
was intubated."

I asked him about last night's echo and Dr. Dubois's suspicions of a clot in the pericardial sac.

"We're going to watch it aggressively. There are no visible strands in the pericardial fluid which would lead us to believe constrictive pericarditis was beginning."

As he talked, Danny made a pumping fist with one hand and overlapped his other hand around this "heart" to act out the feared scenario. By tensing his overlapping hand and tightening its grip on his pumping fist, he graphically showed me the concept of constrictive pericarditis.

"Right now, heart function still looks okay."

Danny sat quietly for a moment more beside us. Some of the brooding look came back into his dark eyes. Something fundamental was bothering him. I had the impression it was Danny's overall assessment of Damion.

"You know, I just don't feel like I have a firm grip on this yet. More than anything else for him, I want to get my belt around this disease." His frustrated hands demonstrated an encircling motion in the soundless air. "I won't be happy until I cinch the buckle shut. I need to lock the first notch in place."

SUNDAY NOON

Having Danny back sped up the pace of decisions. By lunch Damion was cut loose from another lifeline: his dialysis machine. The stump of the catheter implanted into his abdomen was capped off, washed down with Betadine, and the ugly area redressed to guard against infection. No one felt confident enough about his renal situation to consider removing it yet. It was a good thing to keep in reserve.

During lunch Marnix and I talked about the progress of the last twenty-four hours, in terms of measuring improvement by the number of machines supporting Damion. "He's hanging in there without the respirator. He's untied from dialysis. Danny's cranking up his nutrition. This is good progress, despite Danny's general feelings of frustration."

"Mary, how would you feel if I left for a couple of days now that Danny's here? I talked with Danny about it and he saw no imminent reason not to at this point. I could check in on the other children and get a couple of days work behind me. Or you could go, if you want to be home for a few days. What do you want to do? You want to fly home tonight and see the children?"

"Whoa. I never even considered either one of these possibilities."

His words reminded me how differently my husband and I could think sometimes. "If this is some kind of a plateau we've come to, if Danny thinks one of us can go a few days, then I can see the sense in it. But I couldn't leave him now. There's no way I could be useful anywhere else. If I were home, I'd just be preoccupied with how to get back here the soonest way possible."

I was unprepared for this entire conversation and idea.

"The good thing is that whichever one of us goes, with the direct flight to Tallahassee we can be back here in four to six hours," Marnix went on. I knew what he meant: if Damion took another dive, there'd be a way to return quickly.

"I can't leave him," I said slowly. "I can't even imagine what it would be like to leave him. And if it has to be one of us, it may as well be the one who can perform the most functions while they're gone. You can see the children, talk with them about this, and try to make some sense out of the mess I'm sure this has made of your office. You go."

"You don't mind?"

"I don't think so. But I don't know. I've never had the actual experience of being alone here before to know, other than that first day at the first hospital, and I don't expect anything like that could ever happen again. Listen, I think it's okay. I don't feel like it's the wrong idea for right now."

"Okay. Then I'll go, with the understanding that you'll call me every few hours to tell me what's going on. I'm going to have to show you a systematic way of writing down all his vital signs and lab work for me. I'm sure the nurses will keep giving them to you whether I'm here or not. And Danny will continue to involve you."

"Okay. Well, this will be weird without you here for a few days. Why don't you make it as late as reasonable this evening, okay? And you're going to talk to D. about it, right?"

"I know."

SUNDAY AFTERNOON

I sat with Damion alone while Marnix was making arrangements for returning home for a few days. He was muted, very detached again. Danny looked up from his desk and saw that Damion had awakened. Some of Danny's anger was back. It was palpable in the way he asked Damion questions as he stood over the bed, conversational questions like, "Damion, do you want to raise the back of your bed so you can sit more upright for a little while?" Or, "When the nurse brought you that Sprite earlier, how much did you drink?"

When Danny went away, Damion was still connected, determined to reach the goal of having the respirator tube out on Wednesday, still talking to us with his eyes and scribbling notes. Now he was flaccid, depleted, emaciated, a shell of what he was even a week ago. Compared to two weeks ago, or beyond that three when he was still hiking in the woods, Damion was barely recognizable.

I felt Danny's anger. Was it frustration? Or was it a strategy? He walked over to the bin of toiletries and dug in them. He found a comb and threw it on the bed where it landed at Damion's blanketed feet.

"Damion, comb your hair! You look terrible. Now you comb your hair and fix yourself up a bit," he said firmly. Then he turned and strode out of the room.

Damion was shaken. I was surprised. A guilty silence hung between us. After a few minutes, I got up. "I'd better see if Dad needs anything." Damion said nothing. I left through the first set of wooden doors on Damion's side of the unit so I wouldn't have to walk in front of Danny's desk.

When Marnix and I returned a half hour later we found a poignant sight. Damion had somehow scooted the comb up with his feet to where he could reach it. He must have dipped it into a cup of melted ice on the table that was a full stretch from his bed. He had to get water somewhere because his hair was still damp where he had tried to part it. He slept soundly again, but the comb was tucked by his side, under his sheet.

SUNDAY LATE EVENING

"Damion, I'm going to be back soon. It will probably be on Wednesday. Mama's going to call me all the time to tell me how you're doing. Momma can even get a phone put in here so you and I can talk to each other directly.

"I'm going to miss being right here with you but this will be a very short trip. And you know I wouldn't go if you weren't doing so much better now. I'm very proud of you. Just look at what you've been able to do in the last few days: you're off the respirator, off the dialysis machine and one of your chest tubes is out."

"And my oxygen is up to ninety-five," Damion interrupted, proudly pointing to the white light on the overhead monitor.

"That's right, angel. And that's all on your own, with no machine helping you to breathe. You're the one who did all that." Damion looked more confident this evening. He didn't seem distressed that his dad would be leaving in a few minutes. He and Danny had a nice talk alone this afternoon before Danny left for the night. Damion was beginning to show some signs of interest again in what was going on around him, although he still looked very sleepy.

"D.D., I love you. I'd better go or my cab won't wait. But you know I love you, big boy. You be tough till I get back Wednesday afternoon, okay?"

"Okay. Say hi to Sebastian and the little kids for me."

After Marnix kissed Damion goodbye, I walked with him down to the front entrance.

"This is harder than I thought," he said.

In the lobby he stopped and asked me to pull the list out from my pocket again. Marnix had gridded out little squares for each four-hour period from Sunday night to Wednesday afternoon. My job was to record everything within those times and keep him informed.

"You know I'll have my car phone with me all the time so you can get me on that or the pager number."

We started to walk out to the waiting taxi as I continued to read the list aloud.

"You've got a lot to do, Mary."

"I'll try not to screw it up. And you'll be talking with Danny."

Marnix threw his carry-on into the taxi and bent down to hug me.

"Get home safely," I said. "Then hurry back."

"You call me if you need to."

"Yes, dear. I love you. He's going to be all right, don't you think? Or else you wouldn't be going?"

The cab pulled off before he lowered the window. He only had time to say goodbye with his worried eyes.

SUNDAY NIGHT

Sometimes a Dr. Rosenberg came into the unit to man the desk, particularly at night. He was very quiet and barely interacted with us. He remained absorbed in the papers on his desk. It was almost like he was using this time to study, I thought, remembering some of the moonlighting jobs Marnix took during his residency to pay for his apartment and car. I never said more than "Hi" to him as I passed by or heard more than "Hi" back. He struck me as rather impersonal, and I asked one of the nurses what his role was.

"He's a pulmonologist. He helps out with Danny and Dr. Sastry's practice."

"Oh."

But tonight Dr. Rosenberg seemed to have sprung into action. He stayed on the phone in animated conversations that had the urgency of lining up people for an emergency situation. The nurses were also very active, taking things in and out of an unoccupied cubicle beside Damion's. A shortwave radio crackled occasionally, a sound I had never heard in the unit. There were preparations being made.

Soon I learned why. I overheard Dr. Rosenberg instructing loudly on the telephone, "No. I don't even want him up here before he goes to Radiology. Don't you send him up here without a CAT scan series or he'll be going right back down, and we'll all waste time."

"A baby's coming in," Damion's nurse told me quietly when she saw my awareness of the commotion. "It's going to get busy around here."

Within a half hour, paramedics and police burst into the unit, rolling a little stretcher ahead of them. Nurses and Dr. Rosenberg jumped up and crowded around. Someone's arm held up an IV line, and someone else was pushing a cart with equipment and hoses that connected to a mask over the baby's face.

"Let's get him in there!" The stretcher jerked closer toward our space and was quickly driven into the adjacent corner room. Our nurse had left us during this flurry of activity, and now some-one's hand reached in and turned our blinds to a closed position and slid the door shut.

"Good," I thought. I didn't want to see what was happening there. Please just let this little baby be okay, God, I prayed. Please make everything okay.

There were too many voices and too much disruption to think of getting up and going to my room. The closed door was a message, perhaps: Everyone not involved in this, stay where you are. I thought I might be under an unspoken command to do just that. Damion was sleeping and the clock showed that it was after eight. Feeling trapped, wondering what to do until I'd be able to slip out, I picked up Damion's unused CD player, put in my own disk by a haunting Gaelic singer, Enya, and sat down in the more comfortable of the two chairs.

Mournful music, baleful ballads mostly, but very beautiful, very ethereal, played. Closing my eyes and being in the music was the only escape I'd discovered since being thrown into this hard edged world.

After a long interlude, I felt the nurse coming back into our space. I removed my earphones and nodded to her. She was distant and distracted. She went mechanically through some of her tasks with Damion.

"Well, listen," I said wearily. "You know where to find me. I think I'm going to get out of your way and get a few hours of sleep myself." I got up. "Can you tell me one thing? Is the baby going to be okay?"

"No."

She sniffled and kept her eyes on the charting. "His CAT scans are hopeless."

I knew and she knew she had said too much. But she was not only sad but angry about something.

"I'm really sorry. Thank you for looking after Damion tonight. I'm glad you're with him."

As I left the unit, calm had replaced the frenzy of an hour ago. Dr. Rosenberg was staring at cranial x-rays so intently that I escaped to the hall without his even noticing me.

But I found the commotion had simply spilled out there. Between the swinging doors and my room, there were ten to fifteen people standing and watching a dramatic scene unfolding. Two police officers had a man pinned up against the wall near my parent room door. They stood very close to him in a challenging and assertive posture. The young man was no older than twenty-two or twenty-three. The legs of his jeans were torn and ragged. He had a pack of cigarettes in his hand and kept his eyes on them as he fingered them longingly. His expression gave me the impression his biggest problem was that he desperately needed a smoke in a place where no smoking was allowed. The hall crackled with anger and confrontation.

"Excuse me. Is it a problem if I go in there?" I asked an officer close to the doors. "That's my room they're standing in front of."

"Hang back here just a minute, ma'am. I think they're about done."

I joined the assembly of people waiting for some kind of resolution to the tension. Leaning up against the wall, I looked down. In a minute or so, I heard the low voices of the police beside my door coming closer. The people around me started to tense in readiness. Two officers, one on either side of the young man, whose face was now set in defiance, held their prisoner's elbows. As they passed, I saw that handcuffs locked the nervous hands and the cigarette pack was gone. Then the hall emptied and I made it to my room.

"God, I hate this world," I spat out finally free of whatever this new evil was about. I kicked off my shoes, thinking of how far along Marnix might be on his trip by now. I wished he were here to talk with me about what was going on tonight in the unit. He'd help me see it in some kind of perspective. Marnix was good at accepting the complexity of good and evil in life, whereas I found certain things unacceptable and unfathomable. I railed against injustice as though my refusal to accept it could make a difference. He was much more like the Dutch in his approach to iniquity. Not accepting it, not tolerating it, but aware of it and not perplexed by it when he stumbled upon it. It was a mind set I didn't have.

After a quick shower and brushing my teeth, I settled into

bed. Now the emptiness of the room confounded me. I looked at Marnix's clothes and books stacked neatly under his bed. Leaving my bed, I jumped into his, turning on the television on my way across the room. Nothing but the ten o'clock news was on, and I really didn't want to hear it. I switched quickly from channel to channel, but three words from an announcer suddenly stopped my surfing:

"St. Joseph's Hospital."

I turned up the sound.

"Fifteen-month-old Jimmy Brooks was transferred to St. Joseph's with head injuries. The mother's twenty-year-old boyfriend is being questioned by the police." Behind the newscaster was the heading "Child Abuse" on a board.

Oh my God. The little boy fighting for his life, sleeping next door to my boy, is there because someone beat him, I thought. We're there because of an evil bacteria, and he's there because of an evil person. It was incredible really. While we were doing everything we could to save our child's life, Jimmy's family did something to end his.

It was unfathomable and absolutely unacceptable.

14

Sudden Acceleration

"Hey, can I ask you something?"

The father of the little boy who'd been a drowning victim stood outside the doors of the intensive care unit.

"Sure." I tried to smile. "I haven't seen you in a while. How's he doing?"

Boo Man's dad looked terrible. He looked like he'd gotten no sleep since he brought his son in. His brown eyes were circled with the same darkness into which his wife had sunken earlier.

"Well, what I need to know is, do you know anything about this Dr. Plasencia that's come to the unit? We were used to Dr. Sastry, who's taken really good care of him. But now this new doctor is telling me he may have permanent brain damage. He put him on all these machines, and it's going downhill fast."

The young father started to cry, and I knew I couldn't say anything to make him feel better.

"I can't tell you anything about your son, but I can swear to you and so can my husband that Danny's the best thing Boo Man has going for him. He's an unbelievably fine doctor, the best one you could have fighting for your boy."

"He's really okay?"

"Not just okay. Superb."

I gave him a hug and said, "It hurts so badly. I know it. Boo Man needs you and your wife fighting for him. You have to cry but you have to fight like hell, too."

He was a nice man. I felt sad that there was nothing I could do for him.

Hell was breaking loose on our side of the unit when I walked in. A vigil had been set up around baby Jimmy. He lay on his back connected to a respirator with his arms outstretched on IV boards. A circle of teenage girls surrounded the crib. A photograph of Jimmy on the wall over his head showed a beautiful little boy, round, fat, bald, and laughing. Now the lullaby he heard was from this chorus of loudly weeping girls. I couldn't tell which one was the mother. The one that stood with her back to me had on tight jeans and a blue sweater, and none of the girls could ever be described as wholesome, but there was no mistaking the depth of their grief.

One of the nurses was sliding their door shut as I passed. Her face looked angry. Damion's nurse Jane was also somber when I entered Damion's space.

She said, "Please slide the glass shut. It's awful out there."

I turned to my son. "Hi, Damion! You've got only me this morning, but I just talked to Dad and he asked me to ask you to tell me all your monitor numbers." I added as I kissed him, "You smell good!"

"Bathed and ready to go!" Jane bragged.

"Why didn't you guys wait for me?"

"Because Damion woke up early, and we wanted something to do."

"Oh, well." I pretended to be disappointed for Damion's sake. He was tuned in enough to try and entertain.

"So, D., help me fill out this list for Dad. You know what a slave driver he is. And, Jane, can I bother you for the morning labs if they're back yet?"

"I'll get them for you."

"Damion, what's up? Are you having a harder time breathing?"

"A little bit."

I looked at Damion more closely. He was breathing more heavily but he was alert and oriented. He read off his blood pressure, heart rate and oxygen saturation to me as I wrote. He seemed more connected than in previous days, but his nostrils flared as he talked.

"Thanks, buddy. They all sound good. Dad's going to be happy. And I'll get the rest from Jane."

Danny returned to the unit from the other side. He was engrossed in several calls, so I decided to talk to him later. Jane

returned with the lab printout labeled "Hematology," and I began
to copy the numbers for Marnix's grid marked Monday.

"Damion, holy cow! Your platelets are one-ninety-eight this
morning. This is a great jump. I'm so proud of you for getting them
back up there and for knowing so much about all this. John Kelton's
going to kiss you."

Damion smiled.

"I think Danny wants to talk to you," Jane said.

I got up quickly and walked toward the elevated desk. I was
happy about his numbers, but I wanted to know what was wrong
with Damion's breathing.

"It worries me, too," Danny said. He swiveled his chair to the
wall and put up Damion's chest films.

"They look the same," I said, "except maybe more enlargement in the heart, but I can't tell. Is it bigger?"

"Yes. I am concerned that this is going on too long without
improvement. It can be very dangerous."

"I'm calling Marnix with all the statistics this morning. What
do you want me to tell him?"

"Tell him I'm calling orders for another echo and that Dr.
Brodsky and I will call him as soon as we have something definite."

I changed the subject. "And, Danny, I want to thank you for
being firm with Damion when you came back. I don't know how
you did it, but he seems to be pulling out of a depression he had
fallen into."

Danny smiled faintly.

"He's doing better with that aspect. He's been through a lot,
but we can't afford to have him feel defeated. A good attitude men-
tally is very important. We need him fighting again."

Realizing how extremely busy Danny was and that Marnix
wouldn't be able to concentrate on his own patients until he heard
from me, I left to call in the numbers.

Maria, the woman who cleaned the unit, was vacuuming our
room when I entered to use the phone. She turned off the vacuum
and said to me conspiratorially, "You know Baby Jimmy's mama,
they take another child away from her."

Maria had very keen ears. The first times I'd seen her, she

discreetly came in and mopped under Damion's bed and didn't betray the fact that she was listening. But soon she started winking at me in the hallway and making comments like, "We off the ventilator today, no? Dees is good! First time, ten days!"

I got the impression that this compact little woman from Honduras was more tuned into life in the hospital than anyone might expect. She was very sneaky and a stealthy gossip and a well-intentioned spy.

"I come all alone from my conetry," she told me. "But now I have very nice hosband, very good son. I very happy in my work. You need more towels? I get you towels."

"No, you're very kind, but you make me feel guilty when I can get them from the linen cart myself. You spoil me too much."

"Well, she have two more and now they take away. Boyfriend, he do it, but mother very bad to leave baby with monster like heem."

"Maria, how do you know all this?"

"Last night, nurses very mad. They say what police say. Boyfriend have party and baby no stop crying. He throw baby like doll at wall. You see head?"

"Yes."

"My son I love very much. I work very hard for heem. How can people no love their cheeldren?" Maria looked as though she could start to cry.

"I don't know, Maria. Some people in our society are selfish and sick. There are more and more people who don't take care of their children. It's like our culture has gone insane. It's scary. Very scary."

Despite all the good news about Damion, the bad news about his heart worsened. Rather than retreat and move on to hit the next organ system, H.U.S. had dug in on its attack on Damion's heart and lungs. Diversionary tactics and taps would no longer hold back its assault. A direct and dramatic rescue mission was now the only choice. So Dr. Brodsky called in a Dr. Angell.

Dr. Angell's report described the problem and included a plan for surgery to provide a pericardial window and drainage of the pericardium and left pleural space. He discussed with me the operative procedure and the risks and alternatives. The plan was to proceed with the surgery tomorrow morning.

MONDAY NOON

"So they talked with you directly, even Dr. Angell?" Marnix asked when I called him.

"Yes."

Marnix's clipped tone displayed his own distress.

"We don't have much choice, do we?" I asked.

"None."

"So you've managed to be home less than seventeen hours before we call you back. What time will you come in? I'll pick you up at the airport."

Suddenly Marnix veered off the topic of Damion's impending heart surgery and his return. "I got a phone call a few minutes ago," he said. "You know how we've talked about the doors that open as other doors slam shut?"

"Yes."

"You know the Wilson brothers? Their kids go to school with ours? Steve wants to ask you something. He'll call you in the unit in a minute."

"Marnix," I said, my own frustration surfacing. "I've got thousands of things about Damion to think of right now, one of them being when to come get you tonight. Can't you tell me what this is about?"

"No, I want you to talk to him. We'll work out me getting down after that."

"All right, Marnix. Just get here soon, please. I can't get through this evening alone."

"We'll talk in a half hour, Mary."

"Okay, I'm going to sit with Damion and pretend everything is going to be perfectly fine. It's unbelievable. Three hours ago I thought that we'd had a breakthrough, and then I saw him struggling for air again."

"Call me in a half hour."

"Okay. All right, Marnix."

MONDAY AFTERNOON

Damion was still awake. I was glad he was able to stay up longer but wondered if he was having a hard time drifting off because of his difficulty breathing. Or maybe he was worried about

Dr. Angell's plan for him. But I was there at the time, and Damion was informed and involved in the most sensitive way.

"It will be just like a window, Damion," Dr. Angell had explained. "I'll be opening up a small window in the lining of your heart. It will be like letting fresh air in and allowing the junk and fluid trapped inside to escape. You'll be sound asleep, and everything will be okay. When you wake up, you'll be on the respirator a few hours, and then you can come back up from my part of the hospital by late afternoon."

"What's your part called?"

"C.I.C.U. Cardiac Intensive Care Unit."

"And I have to go back on the respirator?"

"Just until you're stable. Probably only a few hours after surgery."

I was impressed with the way everyone here explained things to Damion. It helped him with his fear, and it helped me with mine. Dr. Angell soon left, but Danny sat with Damion and made sure any other questions were answered and that he understood what would happen tomorrow.

Now, I sat beside him glad for the few minutes to be quiet together and alone after the frenetic morning.

Jane tapped me on the shoulder. "Mary, there's a call for you. Someone named Steve Wilson. Do you want to take it?"

"Thank you, Jane," I said, unable to muffle the deep sigh which escaped me.

Steve Wilson sounded far away. I had never spoken with him on the phone before, only seen him in Wilbro's discount store he and his brother George owned in our town. We got all our toys there, for one thing. Sometimes we'd go in on a rainy day to look and come out with things like play houses and Mack trucks.

"I called Marnix earlier and told him that we'd thought of something that might help," Steve said. "I understand you haven't seen your other kids in more than two weeks now, and that must be hard on them and you. You know we have a corporate plane and a pilot who can fly them down and then bring them right back after a visit with you and Damion."

"Oh! Steve, I can't even think about how wonderful that would be."

"We'll do it today. Annette and I can get them out of school and arrange it. The children can be there in a couple of hours and back in their own beds tonight."

"Your timing is incredible. Did you know that Damion's scheduled to have cardiac surgery tomorrow morning?"

"Marnix told me a little while ago." I could feel the slight stirring of air one feels when a door opens.

"Steve, I think it will be a real lift for Damion to see his brothers and sister before he goes into surgery. This is an incredible offer. I'll never be able to thank you enough."

"We just want to help. Okay, it's done. I'll get our pilot to call the hospital late this afternoon and tell them what time he'll be bringing Marnix and the kids into the private airstrip at Tampa Airport."

"Steve, thank you. Thank you all so much," I said, trembling with gratitude.

MONDAY EVENING

Marnix and the children were getting in at 7:15. Determined to meet them at the airport myself, I told Damion that I'd be back within an hour. He was very excited about them coming and had slept hardly at all since he'd found out.

"Damion, they won't get in for another hour, but I'd better go now so I can find the right part of the airport and everything. You stay put," I added jokingly. "Don't take off on me."

He smiled back.

The parking deck beside the hospital complex had four levels, one indistinguishable from the other, and they were all jammed for visiting hours.

As I walked from the lobby and entered the bottom parking deck, I hesitated. I'd gone blank. I couldn't remember was the van on the bottom level, or had I driven up the ramps twelve or thirteen days ago when I was hurrying back from visiting Sebastian? Where had I put the van? "I know the spot was covered, so it wouldn't be on the roof level," I murmured.

I began to search up and down the aisles of the ground level. There must have been a hundred cars, and it took ten minutes. Then I began on the second layer, popping in and out of aisles and seeing if a blue Dodge Caravan stuck out anywhere. By now I had wasted more time than I had to spare. When I reached the third level, I became more frustrated when I saw this too was full. I searched for the van, fuming. I was going to be late. Thinking I hadn't checked the second level thoroughly enough, I rushed down the steps to check again. Maybe I had pulled in so tightly that the rear of the van didn't stick out.

"How could I have lost our van? How could I not remember where I parked it?" I ran back to the third level and searched again. No blue van with Alabama plates.

I sat down on the curb. Maybe what was happening with Damion was not an isolated event in my life. Maybe our whole structure was unwinding—all the big and little elements. Maybe the whole construction of my life was coming to one colossal unraveling. Maybe nothing was possible anymore. A heart that constricted and a memory that froze.

I crouched down on the curbside and cried over my lost car and my misplaced life. And then as the worst pounding of my head stopped, I realized all this was doing no good but only making matters worse.

I rose and took the stairwell down to the ground level and found a little glass office near the entrance and told the security guard my plight. He got on his radio, and soon a vehicle like a golf cart arrived from another hospital parking lot. The driver, a ruddy-complected, gray-haired man, invited me to get in beside him, and we began to drive up and down the aisles I'd just walked through.

"I feel so stupid," I said.

"Why are you so sure you didn't park on the rooftop?"

"Well, I remember it was a hot day, and I thought to myself as I locked the van that at least I had found a covered space."

He grinned suddenly and swung the cart up the ramp to the roof. The sky was darkening as we pulled onto the open deck. I saw immediately a whole line of cars parked under a sheltering overhang.

"There it is! Part of the roof is covered! Listen, I feel like an idiot. I'm sorry for taking your time."

"That's okay. I do this all the time for folks."

Probably just for amnesia victims, I thought. He stayed until

I opened the van and got the motor started, which luckily hadn't run down in the last two weeks. I rolled down my window.

"Thanks! Sorry!"

He smiled. "You sure you know your way to the airport?"

"Yes. Here's my map." I held up the map the nurses had highlighted for me.

He let me go ahead of him down the exit ramps so I could start making up the lost time.

It was a good map. Jane's yellow marker highlighted the route for me. In only fifteen minutes I was entering Tampa Airport and easily found the lane to the private airfields that corporate and charter flights taxied onto. The private airport terminal was an unconventional building. It was a giant tent hanging from suspension poles. It was lit up from within and resembled something between a grounded kite and a Chinese lantern that had landed on its side in the darkness.

When I got into the lobby, I was surrounded by quiet. Enormous tropical plants in glazed tubs guarded the door.

At the information area I learned that the plane coming from Dothan was in the final approach and would taxi right up to the building within five minutes.

Outside, I searched the sky for the lights of the small plane. Where are you, family? Which part of the sky will you descend from? Come and help Damion. Give him the encouragement he needs for tomorrow. Come and make a difference.

At last the plane descended, touched down, and rolled close, finally taxiing to a stop no more than twenty yards away from me. The propellers slowly stopped. I remained up against the shadow of the building. "I'll wait here until I see them come out," I murmured. I had the strangest reluctance to step out toward them. I wanted to see them first. I'd rather watch them without their seeing me. I was almost nervous to see them, almost scared to see my own children! I couldn't begin to figure out why I didn't want to run out to the plane and sweep them up.

The pilot swung the door open and released the folding steps. When all was ready, a small, shy figure came out. It was Bayne. He hesitated at the top of the steps, apparently blinded by the bright light that was focused on the side of the plane. I saw his confused face searching the darkness around him. He timidly stepped down. Then Mila appeared, in her best red dress. She too paused for an instant and then cautiously followed Bayne. Lastly, Sebastian came out, looking lost as he descended.

Then Marnix bent through the door carrying the same bag he had thrown into the taxi last night. He reached the tarmac and collected the children. I was still frozen by the sight of them all, strangely reticent to call out to them. They all looked so big, so young, so lost, so different, so everything to me. Marnix led them to the entrance. Finally they saw me, and we ran toward each other.

Oh, what foreign creatures they'd become in the last seventeen days! As we hugged each other and I held them one at a time, I was sure they couldn't be mine. They were too big. They were too robust. Bayne and Mila's bodies were round, unlike Damion's frail form in the unit. Their knees and elbows were submerged in layers of flesh. Their faces had full cushioned cheeks. They were never this big before. They couldn't possibly be so strong and healthy.

Sebastian stood sinewy against me, put his powerful hand on top of my head, looked down into my face, and said, "Hi, shorty." How can this be? How can he have grown taller since I saw him last? All of this seemed an illusion and yet was reality.

Marnix and I walked behind the children after our round of hugs and hellos. They were eager to look inside the building.

"Marnix, look at them move! I can't believe how strong and nimble they are! They're so agile, but huge!"

"I know. I know what you're saying. When I went home last night and found them safe and strong in their beds, I had the same reaction. It's a matter of contrast."

"They're so healthy. Look at them move!"

My own children were astonishing to me. They were absolutely wonderful to watch as they raced into the building, yanked on the heavy glass doors, trampled into the cool lobby, and swiftly tried out every seat in the space while we talked briefly with the pilot who had come up behind us. I didn't listen as Marnix lined up what time they'd be back. I couldn't take my eyes off these hardy, active children. They were impossibly vigorous, impossibly mine.

On the way to the van, Mila hugged me again.

"I missed you, Mom."

I stopped, lifted her off her feet, and held her roundness to me. Her fleshiness was a treasure against my body!

"And I missed you so much, too, baby girl. I'm so glad you're here. Damion can't wait to see you. Thank you for coming!"

MONDAY NIGHT

During the elevator ride up to the eighth floor, Marnix reminded the children how to behave in the intensive care unit. "Now," he said, "you know what we talked about. You have to be quiet and in control in there. And remember that Damion will be weak now. He might get tired easily and can't take a lot of excitement. Don't forget how I told you we all need to wash our hands in the sink inside the door. I'll show you how."

As I led them into the unit, Jane called out, "Hey, everybody, come and see! These are Damion's younger brothers and sister!"

Three nurses popped their heads out of their cubicles and smiled. Two more came out of the supply room with Terri.

"You all look alike!"

"Wow, you kids sure look like a family all right."

"Damion sure has missed you guys!"

The nurses were anything but quiet as we all trooped in to see Damion. I couldn't resist nudging Marnix. His admonishments to be quiet were overridden by the nurses' enthusiasm that Damion's family was here to see him.

Bayne, Mila, and Sebastian looked furtively around at all the equipment and glassed spaces. They saw baby Marty kicking his feet in the air, the comatose Jimmy, and a nine-year-old girl who had recently been admitted. I remembered my own first impression of the unit and thought it must seem like outer space to them. They answered the nurses' pleasant questions and reverently took in the surroundings until Terri said, "Well, get in there. You didn't come to see us. Damion's waiting for you!"

It was so great to be together! They walked up to Damion gingerly, looking as much at his tubes and monitor as they did at him, and then they began speaking softly as Marnix had instructed. Marnix and I smiled to see that Damion had put on his glasses, combed his hair, and pulled the sheet way up against his chin. They couldn't see the chest tube, the dressings over his heart from the taps, the wire threaded into his skin under his collar bone, or any of the offensive catheter lines.

Marnix and I sat in the chairs and let them interact. We listened to the questions they asked Damion and his answers about the monitor numbers, the E.T. light, the IV, and the upside down bottle of white lipids. It was a matter-of-fact discussion, and eventually they ran out of questions. Silence filled the room as they awkwardly looked down at him. Damion pushed up his glasses, waiting for another question. Then Mila obliged.

"So, Damion, how does it feel to be almost dead?"

"Mila!"

Aghast, Sebastian and Bayne reacted. Sebastian elbowed her sharply.

Damion just blinked his eyes, now knowing what to say.

"Well, I just wanted to know."

I had to dive in and rescue this one, I thought. So I tried.

"I know what Mila means. She wants to know how it felt when Damion was very sick over the last two weeks, while he was in a lot of danger. Now that he's getting better and the doctors know how to fix his heart tomorrow so he can finish getting all the way better, she probably just wants to know how it felt to be as sick as he was."

Damion seemed reasonably satisfied with this explanation, and Mila was astute enough to know when to back off. I knew what she meant, and she knew what she meant, but she now realized by everyone's reaction that her real question couldn't be answered.

Just then Marnix picked up a Polaroid camera. "All of you line up on one side of the bed," he said. Damion pushed up his glasses that kept falling down his thin face.

"Children, we are so glad to be together again, thanks to Steve and George Wilson. Let me see a good smile from all of you." Marnix snapped the picture. "Okay, one more."

After a little while Damion showed signs of tiring. He was growing out of breath. Watching his siblings and hearing their chatter had become too exhausting.

"Take a rest, Damion," I said. "Dad and I will take the children downstairs to eat and then they can come back to say good night before I drive them to the airport."

In the cafeteria we ate a family meal, more or less. It was strange but wonderful to be together. No one spoke much of the changes they'd seen in Damion moments before. It seemed to have helped them to actually see him. Watching them eat spaghetti and hearing them talk about the flight down, I realized how beautifully resilient children were. They had seen Damion, they had asked what they needed to know, they'd taken the uncertainties on faith that he would get better, and they seemed okay with it. How could Marnix and I ever hope to recapture their kind of trust and acceptance, I wondered.

Marnix looked at his watch.

"Guys, it's time to say good night to Damion, and the pilot's expecting you back in half an hour. We'd better head on up to Damion's room now."

The children cleaned the spaghetti sauce stains from the tabletop. Napkins piled on their plates looked like they'd mopped up cups of it. Their drinking glasses had traces of it smeared around the bases.

Had they always been so messy at the table? If they were, I'd forgotten that part, too.

As their plane ascended into the sky, I watched the lights until the hazy cloud cover absorbed them. "There go my other children. There they go away again. I don't know when I'll see them. No one knows if Damion will ever say good night to them again."

As I passed under the sentinel plants at the terminal door, I left without knowing which particular sadness or fear caused the tears which fell from my eyes.

TUESDAY MORNING, MARCH 17

When the alarm rang in the dark room, I knew I woke to the worst dread that I could ever imagine.

Oh, it's today! It's going to be this morning! No one can stop it from being today.

We wanted to spend as much time with Damion as possible

before he was scheduled for Dr. Angell's second surgery of the day. Marnix spoke to me in the dark, giving me assurances from his own experience.

"It's good to be the second surgery."

His voice was definitive and confident.

"If you're the first surgery, it's possible the surgeon isn't loosened up or even awake yet. And you never want to be one of the later cases when doctors start to get tired. Number two is just about where you want to be on the schedule. It's as close to ideal as you can get."

"Marnix, tell me one more time. Why is this a good thing?"

"Because he needs it. It's good because it will fix something which is broken."

"Okay, I understand that. I know that. So this is going to be a good thing," I said to myself a thousand times between then and the time they came for him two hours later.

"This will be a good thing."

But the good thing did not start with a good omen.

At 5:30 I walked alone into the unit. Marnix always managed to beat me there by at least five minutes. When I stepped into the unit and looked around, I knew it had happened. Baby Jimmy had died while we slept. His cubicle was empty and scrubbed clean. It showed no trace that he had ever been there, living out the last thirty hours of his life in this room next to Damion's. The sterile space was not the sort of place a little spirit might linger.

The nurse at the desk saw me look into his space.

"Three-thirty this morning," she whispered mournfully.

Her reddened eyes showed that she had cried. The initial rage that none of the staff could hide the night Jimmy came in had deepened into sorrow over the four nursing shifts that he survived.

The doctors and nurses had tried so hard to save him as they tried so hard to save all who came there. It was the unifying principle of everything they did. They were incredibly devoted and committed to their mission. A criminal case of abuse like baby Jimmy put an impossible demand upon them. How could they so fiercely try to uphold a life, when someone else so casually destroyed it? They were left to pick up the pieces and, failing that, to comfort and love what was left. No matter how much care they summoned up for little Jimmy, in the end, it wasn't enough for the child whom no one had truly loved.

We talked quietly, positively with Damion until they came to take him down. It was a quiet morning in the unit. Soon dawn came. People from the lab started to come into the unit with their caddies of vials and tubes and needles. Danny came in for the day. The phone began to ring more frequently.

At 7:30, Danny stood over the gurney, as the orderlies from cardiac surgery waited for him to release their patient and all the support equipment through the P.I.C.U. doors.

"We'll look after your things while you're gone," Danny promised.

By now the wall in Damion's cubicle was filled with a huge collage of cards and letters and banners and photos. His accumulation of toys and animals and small games from Dothan and his cousins filled the window sill. None of these had been played with, but we kept them there in the hopes that he would eventually feel well enough to want them scattered on his bed.

"You hurry back up to us, okay, Damion?" Danny patted Damion's head before the gurney pushed off through the doors.

We gathered in a little vestibule of sorts, the linoleum passage at the mouth of the operating room. All of us jammed into the space between two sets of swinging doors: the nurses, Marnix and I, Damion on his gurney, and all his monitors and tubes and IV poles. It was a crowded space dense with the intimacy of another goodbye. I kissed his forehead. Marnix whispered reassurances. These were reassurances as much for ourselves as they were for Damion.

Beat the odds, Damion. Fight. Fight back, darling. I know you're very tired. But fight back, D. Please don't quit. Please wake out of the anesthesia. Please wake up for Dad and me.

I silently prayed while I stroked his hair and Marnix leaned over him, telling Damion, "This is going to be fine, this is going to let you get better." We verbalized our hopes but everyone in the crowded space knew his odds were diminishing. Marnix especially knew. Upstairs, Danny knew Damion's odds were less good today. We all knew how compromised Damion already was, how damaged and malnourished and tenuous his condition was going into another surgery.

The doors swung open. On the other side, the gloved hand of a masked anesthesiologist beckoned everyone but Marnix and me into the brilliant fluorescence of the operating room.

"I love you, sweet boy," I managed to say.

"Night-night, big boy," Marnix whispered.

For a long time, Marnix and I stood alone in the vestibule. We didn't know where to go. Stepping back out into the corridor, I saw Dr. Angell approaching from down the hall.

"It's Dr. Angell," I said to Marnix.

Angell strode quickly toward us with the loosened paper of his surgical gown flaring out like blue gossamer wings in his haste.

While Dr. Angell quickly introduced himself to Marnix, I thought about his name. It was a good name for someone who would be cutting open a boy's chest very soon, I told myself. Could there be reassurance in a name? Was this an omen worth trusting?

Dr. Angell began explaining our options about the incision. "Some adolescent patients prefer the incision along the armpit and down the side of the rib cage. Cosmetically, some of them find it easier to live with. Or, we could retract the rib cage and do a straight cut right down the middle of his chest, a sternotomy."

Retracting the rib cage I knew meant spreading it apart with viselike tools.

What a choice! This cold blue angel was extending to us a choice of how we'd prefer Damion to be cut! I could not begin to measure the value of each terrible choice. I was still reeling with the thought of even having such a choice presented.

Thankfully, Marnix asked, "What's the simplest? What involves the least amount of time in surgery?"

Good thinking. Thank you, Marnix. Which would require the least time and the least manipulation for our already depleted child?

Dr. Angell didn't hesitate. "The sternotomy."

"Which will heal more quickly?"

"The sternotomy."

Dr. Angell focused his azure eyes on me. "Let me ask you, Mrs. Heersink. How sensitive do you believe your son will be about his scar?"

In my mind I pictured how Damion would look, but it was impossible. I searched for an image of him swimming. I tried to imagine him running his hands down his inflated chest like wet adolescent boys proudly do when they get out of the water with their friends. How will he think about his body? It was impossible to envision: the picture was blocked. A more important question stood in the way: would he be alive this summer when I took the children to the pool?

"Dr. Angell, I can't imagine him being self-conscious." I stared at the blond hairs on the hands that would do it.

Marnix was deciding now. I could feel him deciding. "Sternotomy. Mary, you agree." Marnix spoke more quietly now, soberly. "Let's limit his time in surgery. Let's limit the degree of manipulation. Let's remember how malnourished and challenged he already is. Let's think about healing more rapidly."

"Sternotomy," I said to Dr. Angell.

"Then that's what we'll do. Now, you know that at this point the plan is to do a window procedure. We'll have to assess once we get in and see the condition of the pericardium. You understand this?"

"Yes." We nodded.

"We anticipate it will be about two hours before you can see him. You can wait in the C.I.C.U. waiting room around the corner. We will call for you once Damion's in recovery."

And with that, the unmerciful angel flew to Damion.

As we started slowly down the hall, I was struck with the contrast of this floor to the pediatrics department upstairs. Everything down here was steeped in seriousness and stress. There was nothing upbeat like the eighth floor's pastels or sights of children's toys. Here, family members walked the halls with most of life's assurances drained out of their faces. The nursing stations maintained far more equipment than the stations on the average hospital floor. Video monitoring screens stood above the nurses' desks. Emergency carts stood ready at several locations.

Peering into patient rooms, I saw old slippered feet on beds and white hair over hunched shoulders. Everyone was old here. What was an eleven-year-old doing on this floor, a kid whose heart was perfection three weeks before?

"What does one do during two hours like these?" I asked Marnix.

"Perhaps we should leave the building and go for a walk," he said.

"Marnix, I don't want to be around anyone. Please don't take me where we have to see people."

"Just a few minutes. We have to get out of here a few minutes."

He pulled me along, into the elevator, through the glass doors, and outside.

A couple of families leaned on the white ramp walls. Little children were pointing and reaching into the shallow cement pool where giant goldfish swam lazily.

I said, "Marnix, do you promise me you believe it's going to be all right?"

"This will be okay. It's almost a mechanical problem and they can fix it. Just force yourself to think of that."

"Tell me how you can have convinced yourself of this. How can you know this will work?"

"It will. I feel it."

"I can't feel it. Or anything about how it will turn out. It's the most extreme thing yet to me. Is it the worse thing that's happened so far? Of course it is."

"They are fixing it. Believe that."

"I'm trying. I'm trying."

This point was unresolvable, so we just walked without talking. We walked and walked pointlessly. Up and down rows of glinting parked cars in the exposed lot. This was a world hardened by sunlight. We held hands and walked through glaring paths of glass, chrome, and glistening colors.

We walked on and on through the heat silently. His throat must be raw, too, I thought as we inhaled the pollen and the exhaust-laden air swirling around us.

"Let's get back."

"No, there's too much time left. You haven't been outside in days, and there's nothing we can do in there. Let's walk around until there's less than one hour left. Okay?"

"God, it's unbearable out here."

"It won't be any better inside."

He was right.

When we went back, we silently waited out the rest of the time in the empty room. Marnix left occasionally to make telephone calls. I could see him through the open door standing at the pay phone down the hall. He's lost a lot of weight, I thought, staring at him. He's far too thin now.

TUESDAY, LATE MORNING

A woman in a pink volunteer's uniform motioned us to follow her to a door labeled C.I.C.U. "If you'll just wait here, the doctor will be out in a minute to talk with you."

Instead of Dr. Angell, a tall, heavy man with curly brown hair and a strong boxy face came out the door. He introduced himself as Dennis Pupello, chief of cardiac surgery. "Damion did all right," he said. Not waiting for our gratitude to be expressed, he went on, "But when Dr. Angell and I saw the condition of his pericardium, we had to abandon the idea of a simple window. You're a physician, are you not?" he asked Marnix. "Very well then. Mrs. Heersink, you let me know if there's something you don't follow."

He took a breath. "The sternotomy was done in the usual fashion, the incision running from sternal notch to xiphoid process. The pericardium was worse than we anticipated. It was reduced to a shaggy, red-gray granular membrane scattered with areas of gray exudate. Unfortunately, we had to do a pericardial strip instead of the window."

I tried to visualize the tattered lining of his heart.

Dr. Pupello looked at me for a moment and then continued. "So the pericardium was excised and stripped. The tissue was very fragile and tore into small fragments as we removed it. We made sure that all the fibrinous exudate was stripped from the heart. Both chests were then drained. We saw quite a bit of effusion in there, but tubes should alleviate most of that.

"He did well under anesthesia. He's now in C.I.C.U. where

we'll keep him until his signs level out. He's got a bit of a temperature and his heart rate's shaken up a bit. We'll have to watch him carefully and hope he can get back upstairs soon."

Marnix asked, "Have the pericardial tissue and fluid been sent for analysis?"

"Oh yes. We'll be getting full cytology and microscopic reports on them. From just a gross diagnosis point of view, I'd describe the fluid as bloody, and the pericardial tissue as fibrinopurulent pericarditis."

"May we go in yet?" I asked.

"Yes, go to him now," Dr. Pupello answered. "I'll be checking on him periodically throughout the day. We'll talk more later if you have questions."

"Thank you, doctor. Thank you for what you've done."

"Marnix, he's still alive," I said when Dr. Pupello left.

I felt relieved, somewhat elated. But when we pushed on the door and entered the Cardiac Intensive Care Unit, I was totally unprepared for what we found. Directly ahead of us was Damion's bed surrounded by banks of machinery and attended by a C.I.C.U. nurse.

Without even an attempt at friendliness, she instructed, "After you scrub your hands, you can stand on that side of the bed for fifteen minutes."

Marnix and I obeyed, staring into the porcelain bowl as we poured disinfectant on our hands. Now our hands were clean and it was time to gather our courage and walk over there and wedge ourselves tightly between the machines and the poles.

Damion lay half naked on an ice water mattress, trembling from the subsiding anesthesia and the trauma of being cut open with a saw. The respirator was the only piece of equipment I recognized. A collection of monitors and machines so numerous that Marnix and I had to take turns standing close to him surrounded our son.

Parents aren't supposed to see their children this way, I thought.

The worst for me was seeing a huge new dressing in the middle of Damion's chest, ten square inches of gauze punctured by a clear tube the diameter of a garden hose. Through it, sticky bloody fluid snaked its way from the deep recesses of Damion's chest to a plastic bag clipped against his bed. Already, it looked like a quart had accumulated.

This is what is drowning you, Damion, this and the same liquid oozing out of your two side drain tubes.

Still I had to calm myself to think of him, to help him.

"Precious boy, Mom and Dad are here."

"He hears you," the businesslike nurse said to us.

I was taken aback by her lack of gentleness. She sat in a manly way, elevated on a stool that swiveled in all directions for access to the monitors and switches around her. I had never seen so much high tech in my life! Even Marnix looked intimidated by it all.

She offered us her clipboard. On it was a sheet with a grossly disfigured scrawl.

"*It is hard to breath.*" Under that, with a balloon drawn around it for emphasis, he had written, "*Can I have a sheet over me,*" and at the bottom of the page, another entry: "*I'm cold. Will you please put the bed on low warm.*"

"He wrote this? Since he's been out of surgery?" I asked, amazed that Damion was so lucid so quickly.

She asked for the pad back, flipped the page, and handed it back for us to read another entry: "*Can they come in now?*"

"We're communicating well with one another," she said abruptly. "I'm Sandy. Watch those lines behind you." She gestured to me. "Step this way a few inches."

I moved away from a tangle of wires and we continued to read the nearly illegible thoughts of our sleeping, shivering Damion.

"*What time is it?*"

"*Can I lie on my left side because it's most comf?*"

"*Last time when I got the tube out they gave me a Popsicle.*"

"I'm taking good care of him," Sandy remarked without looking at us. Instead, she carefully scanned the lights and digital displays behind the head of his bed.

"That's a P.C.A. pump," she said when she saw me looking at an attachment to his left wrist. "Patient-controlled analgesic. Pain pump. It lets him administer his own doses of morphine as he needs them. It's calibrated to limit him to four doses in an hour." I was glad to see he had some degree of control.

"The reason he's sleeping right now is the morphine, not so much the anesthesia."

Marnix asked her about Damion's temperature.

"It was at a hundred and three. That's why he's on the cold water mattress."

More questions about his vital signs.

"Heart rate is up. One-fifties, one-sixty. It's high, which is not unusual after. The same with his elevated blood pressure. That too should come down once his body gets over the shock of the procedure."

She flipped through one of the charts she was keeping on him. "Here are his blood gas numbers. We'll turn the oxygen volume down on the ventilator as his numbers improve."

She described some of the equipment as I kept my hand on Damion's clammy forehead. "It's okay, baby. It's okay," I whispered between the beeps and clicks and deep sighing from the machines that breathed for him, measured him, and watched over all his functions.

I looked around. This was a holding place for patients during the critical post-op phase.

Right beside us was a little five-year-old who preceded Damion in surgery. His mother leaned quietly over him. A few hours later he was moved back to the eighth floor P.I.C.U. because he had done so well. Damion remained in the second floor cardiac intensive care unit.

TUESDAY AFTERNOON

Marnix and I visited Damion frequently, staying for the allotted fifteen minute segments. His nurse Sandy did not strictly enforce this policy, especially when she realized Marnix was an asset for her. I had adjusted to Sandy's manner. She was tough and bossy, but her sense of control was greatly reassuring. I could tell Marnix respected her, and Damion needed her. Even now I felt better about her no-nonsense, take-charge personality.

"All right, Damion. I'm going to disconnect your respirator and suction you out. You're not going to panic about it, are you? You just wait until I count to ten, then I'll plug your hose back in and you'll get air. Got that? Okay, let's do it. One, two, three. . . ."

We knew that she was orchestrating everything for him, and that we were there only to assure him of our presence and not to stay so long that we'd distract Sandy from doing her duty.

Danny came down in the afternoon to visit Damion. "You look pretty good for all you've been through," he said. However, he noted something that Sandy had started to be concerned about also. Damion's red blood count was dropping quickly. They called Dr. Pupello who ordered that they should feed packed red blood cells through his IV. More blood. Again, there was no choice.

TUESDAY EVENING

By dinnertime, Damion was stabilized enough so that we felt we could leave together. We had company. Marnix's brother Hans with his daughter Carine had driven from Canada. Damion and Carine were only a year apart and were good friends and cousins to each other.

Because all four of us would be too many in the unit, the grownups waited in the hall while Carine visited Damion for fifteen minutes. I was certain that seeing Carine would be uplifting. I was sure that he would be glad when she talked to him. But in my focus on what was good for Damion, it hadn't occurred to me how the visit would affect her. Carine looked shaken when she came out of the C.I.C.U. I patted her hand and all of us headed for the cafeteria.

"Carine, I know you helped him by being there."

She had carried a carved wooden giraffe from a souvenir shop at Busch Gardens. "There was no place to put it in there, but I showed it to him. Can you keep it somewhere for him until he has a spot to put it?"

"Good choice in animals." I smiled. "This looks just like the D. After dinner I'll take you up to the intensive care unit where he's decorated his little room with his things. This will be waiting for him on his window sill up there."

"Oh, here are the notes he wrote when we talked. Some are to his nurse and some are to me. Do you want to read them?"

I noticed his penmanship was improving hourly. His letters

now stayed within the lines and punctuation was appearing more frequently.

"Can I have my medicine button?
"Turn down the TV.
"I'm right-handed and I can't reach it with my right.
"I already have lots of unopened things upstairs.
"What flavors of Italian ice do they have?"

"May I keep the paper?" Carine asked as I folded it back up. I could see from her trembling that it was hard for her to be confronted by someone in Damion's condition, especially her cousin. Her own father was shocked at Damion's appearance. How could it not be troubling to a thirteen-year-old? Were Marnix and I becoming so accustomed to the sight of Damion in trouble that we didn't consider his impact on other people who knew him as a big robust kid?

I tried to reassure her. "Carine, you helped D. so much by being with him. Do you know you're the first young person he's seen in weeks, besides last night's visit from his brothers and sister? And you're one of his best buddies. Thank you so much for going in there."

"I'm glad I did." She paused, her voice shaking slightly. "But it was awful."

Despite her words, by now I was feeling better. But I could feel Marnix's growing worry. He was more and more upset about Damion's elevated temperature and heart rate, but Damion had survived this new assault. For this I was very grateful. Still, Marnix brooded about Damion's temperature and heart rate through dinner.

Hans and Carine listened in a subdued mode as he blurted out, "High 150s are much too high. He's going to get worn out. And this fever is not good."

We were going through one of our role reversals. I had been abysmal all morning while Marnix was certain everything would work out. Now I felt inflamed with confidence. I leaned over the table trying to convince these nonresponsive brothers. "But he's alive! He actually came through the surgery. He is living!" And then a few minutes later, "He made it. And you know, Marnix—Hans, you know this—today was his most threatening roller coaster loop yet."

Neither offered any concession to my point. Carine sat there still more or less stunned. Perhaps we should all have been more discreet about involving her.

"Come on, guys. This should be a celebration. This morning I just knew something would crash in surgery and that he wouldn't be here tonight. Please be happy. We should all be encouraged, ecstatic, that he made it."

No one answered. We finished our meal in silence. Marnix and I were polarized at opposing ends of belief and disbelief. Tonight, however, Marnix had his brother and a stunned thirteen-year-old to share his deepening worry. I was left to the lonely celebration of my renewed hope.

When the elevator opened onto the second floor after dinner, we were amazed to find David and Katy Maddox, friends from home, standing outside the C.I.C.U. door. David was the son of a beloved minister and worked with the youth in his church.

"David! Katy! How'd you get here? Oh, it's great to see you both! This is Marnix's brother Hans and his daughter Carine."

We learned that the Maddoxes had taken their children to Disney World and detoured two hours out of their way to visit us. Their children had been on their feet all day at the park and were now asleep in their van under the eye of their thirteen-year-old.

"Will you come and see Damion?" I asked. "He's right inside this door."

Dave and Katy declined. They stood somber. "We've come to be with you." This was disappointing: in my state of euphoria I wanted the whole world to see that Damion was alive.

Marnix told them about the surgery and Damion's status over the last few days. As he talked, David and Katy stood very close to him, mournful looks on their faces.

I wanted to interrupt, *No, you don't understand. You see, Damion is alive tonight. He had a substantial chance of not making it through the day. But now it's night and, on the other side of this door, if you'd just step in, you'd see for yourselves that he is living!*

I didn't say anything as they said goodbye to Marnix who was heading back into the unit with Hans and Carine. Rather, I hopped into the elevator with them and rode down, asking too many questions about Disney World and their three boys. I hardly recognized my own nonstop ebullience. "You're really going to drive all the way home tonight after being at Disney all day? After coming all the way over here?"

I didn't explain that I wanted everyone to celebrate Damion's survival of the day. I didn't express how lucky we felt to still have him. As they said goodbye at the front doors, I wondered if they were perplexed by the dramatic contrast between Marnix's and my emotions. Did they perceive me as manic? Him as depressive? As they walked away, I began to shout after them, "*Hey, Maddoxes! Not so glum, please! He is ALIVE!*"

Was everyone out of synch with reality here? Or was I the inappropriate one, thrilled that my son was in cardiac intensive care, his blood still being pumped by a besieged heart?

WEDNESDAY MORNING, MARCH 18

When we walked in to see Damion I was astonished to find him watching television.

"Good morning, angel."

Marnix and I leaned over Damion and engaged in a conversation that was one way, except for Damion's intermittent nods and squinting eyes. Now I could look at him closely. He appeared comfortable and alert. He was interested in the television mounted overhead. This was one of the few times I was convinced of the value of television. This place, I thought, would be slow torture without the balm of morphine or the numbing opiate of the tube.

Sandy was back again, which was a calming influence on us. She watched over Damion like a hawk. To update us, she handed us the fragments of conversations he had with the late night nursing shift and her earlier this morning. Reading these little penciled wishes was like peering into a window of Damion's confining experience. They let us know what he had struggled with, what his questions were, what he wanted.

We could see the fluctuations in his mood and needs during the shift changes. After Sandy left him last evening, we saw his need to assert himself to her replacement:

"*Earlier when you said 'You won't try to pull your tubes out?' and I said 'no,' I had a tube just like it in P.I.C.U. for a week!!!*

And I got aggravated and annoyed with it but still I lived with it and toughed it out and didn't pull it out."

Later, in the middle of a night which didn't darken for him, because of the fluorescent lights, the new nurse had written "early Wed. A.M." in the margins.

"My right side hurts whenever I breath."

"When am I getting my tube out and my penis tube out?"

"How long will it be after I get the tube out before I can have liquids?"

"What's a blood gas?"

Then we came to a page where Damion's pencilings were interrupted by a penned memo to him from the reappearing Sandy. She had drawn large exclamation points with smile lines under them, pictograms that seemed to say, "I'm back! Now let's get down to business." These bossy little graphics appeared at the beginning and at the end of a memo which read:

THE PLAN
1. MOUTH TUBE OUT
2. (MAYBE) NOSE HOSE OUT (POPSICLE TO FOL-
   LOW)
3. ONE CHEST TUBE DRAIN OUT
4. BLADDER TUBE OUT

Then came the frustrated persistence of a thirsty critically ill boy:

"Can I have some Italian ice like the first time I had my tube removed with my Popsicle?"

"Can you pour Sprite?"

"Am I going back up to my room this mourning?"

"Tell her to reattach me: I can hardly breath!"

"With my head up, I can breath much better."

"Can you turn down the bed temp just a little so that it's cold, but not too cold?"

"What is all the brown stuff coming from my stomach in my nose tube?"

"When I am able to eat, can I have whatever I want?"

"Will you put a cold rag on top of my head and call my parents"

Marnix and I had to reiterate to Damion what Sandy had told him and defer to her when we didn't know the answers to his questions. His notes continued and were mostly about his physical needs. Here and there other elements seeped in:

"You missed it. Jennifer Capriatti beat Monica Seles."

WEDNESDAY AFTERNOON

Unfortunately, the optimistic plan that Sandy had drafted for Damion did not come true. Dr. Pupello came by and noted that the central chest tube was still draining too much fluid. Several liters had gone into the collection bag. The side chest tubes drained as well.

"What would happen if all this was building up in his chest with no way to get out?" I asked Marnix in the cafeteria at noon.

"He'd drown."

I looked away.

Dr. Sastry, or Sid as Damion called him, also came down to check on Damion. He considered all the statistics and made a decision.

"He's not ready to go back upstairs today. With his heart rate, pressures, and the amount of chest drainage he's better off down here for another night. They're better equipped to handle it if anything deteriorates in the night."

It was true that the heart and lung monitoring was more sophisticated than in the P.I.C.U. One nurse to guard him was also a reassurance. But I knew Damion would be unhappy about not being able to go back up to "his room" as he'd come to think of it. How strange for all of us that what was initially so intimidating an environment now felt like home.

WEDNESDAY NIGHT

The roller coaster car was reaching level ground again. Damion's temperature was coming down and staying down more consistently. His heart rate was dropping out of the high 150s and began to stabilize around 140. Marnix was relieved by this evening's report from Bacteriology. The pericardial tissue and fluid continued to show no growth on the lab readouts. These aerobic culture reports were printing out a reassuring negative for the first twenty-four hours.

"That's good. The last thing he needs is some cardio-pulmonary infection cooking up inside him," Marnix repeated to me as we were settling down for bed. "But really, I'm not surprised. This is part of the same edematous process we've seen all along. One organ after another bloating up with this weeping serous fluid. And you know what? If it weren't for the plasma exchange, it would be these same organs one after another taking hits, fatal hits with clots from all the sludge that would have been aggregating in his blood."

We got off easy, I thought sarcastically as he talked. Instead of fluid they could manage with chest tubes and by stripping off his pericardium, we could have been faced with emboli and infarcts to the heart and lungs that would kill critical tissue. Kill him.

At what point do we leave this dangerous stage? I wondered.

Marnix explained the objective from here. "We need to get a few more plasma treatments in, if we can. We want every possibility of more damage blocked off. When we get him upstairs tomorrow, Dr. Rodwig's lining up another exchange. Now I want to continue plasma until John feels absolutely confident that we've done everything we can to avoid any more complications."

"But, Marnix, aren't you so glad he seems to be pulling out of this last loop? Aren't you so grateful that he made it through yesterday's surgery and all this rocky post-op stuff so far? Do you feel better about him tonight?"

He answered, "I'll feel better when we get the lines pulled out of him and he starts having perfectly clear chest x-rays and after one week with no more disasters."

I ventured out onto the ledge of hope. "I think for the first time I'm beginning to think that can happen. For the first time, I think he will make it. Tomorrow, step one: he's upstairs. And that'll be one thing you can check off you list."

"Let's get some sleep," Marnix said, exhausted by the sheer weight of it all.

THURSDAY MORNING, MARCH 19

"<u>MOM!</u>"

It was the written equivalent of a scream, an emphatic seven lines tall consuming the width of the pad which Damion had written angrily during the night.

"D., were you asking for us in the night?"

He nodded his head in a hurt yes.

"I'm sorry, darling. We didn't know."

Sandy was back for the third day. "We took care of it, didn't we, Damion? That was at 5:30 this morning, and I told him you needed your sleep. We solved it on our own."

I looked back at the notes he'd scrawled. They continued:

"Will you go get mom please?

"Did you contact Sid?

"Can I have a bag of ice?

"Why did you say I'm not taking many deep breaths? Saying that will convince them to leave it in another day. I want it out!"

"When today am I going upstairs?"

The notes showed him becoming more and more impatient. Then in tall letters, as if it was his angry way to change the subject, he had written: *"TV REMOTE!"*

Now it was 7:00 A.M. I asked him, "What's up, Damion? Is there anything Mom and Dad can do for you?"

He picked up the pad that was always beside him. I noticed that his hands were very bony. They were becoming the hands of an old man. He seemed about at the end of his rope, totally exasperated with two days and two nights immobilized by monitors and wires and tubes. Looking down, he could watch his bloody chest fluids snake their way out of his wound. He had no privacy, with a nurse two feet away who watched his every sign and movement. He had a fever that wouldn't break. He was not able to wipe away his own sputum. He could not even inhale and exhale when he wanted to. No darkness or quiet to sleep in and an unrelenting pain that only morphine could ease. It was enough to drive anyone over the edge, I thought as I watched my son labor over the angry words.

"When am I getting my tube out? When are they coming?"

Without knowing why, I wrote the response instead of speaking it, maybe for the same reason Sandy wrote down her Plan yesterday.

"Eight o'clock guesstimate, darling. Definitely get you out of here today. The chest tube in the middle has to come out first, and that should be at 7:15 or 7:30."

"How do you know?"

"I was just upstairs with Daddy and Dr. Sastry. They are coming down any minute. Their plan is to free you of the big chest drain so we can move you back up to your room. You're doing better today with your fever and heart rate. Sandy told me you are ready to leave as soon as we unplug you. She told me that Dr. Pupello says so, too."

"And the breathing tube out today, too?"

"That we are not sure about. When you get upstairs, the doctors will take chest x-rays and talk about that. I don't think anyone will be able to make a decision on the respirator until they see the pictures of your lungs, okay? But at least you'll be settled back in your own space today. That's a promise I've heard this morning from Dr. Sastry."

Within an hour and a half, Damion did in fact have the horribly large and ugly chest drain pulled out from his incision. The dressings covering his sternotomy were changed and rebandaged.

"Won't they have to sew that big hole up?" I asked Marnix.

"I don't think so. I believe they'll just tape it closed and allow the tissue to knit back together."

"Good grief, what a big gaping hole it will leave."

"You'd be surprised once they take it out. The opening won't be the width of the tube itself."

"I think I'm more glad than anyone to see this tube go. I just can't get over this huge puncture in his chest. I know it's morbid to think about, but I wonder how deep it extends inside his chest cavity. I try not to think about these things, but it's hard not to when you see that amount of fluid pouring out over the last two days."

"It did its job for him. Try harder not to think about things like that."

"I know. After today, I won't have to. This one is gone."

Soon we were saying farewell and thanking Sandy, who had earned appreciation from all three of us. Marnix respected her commanding competent way. I knew, too, that this was exactly the style of nursing that Damion needed during his stay in C.I.C.U. If you were totally imprisoned within a dangerous situation, it was best to have a benevolent but uncompromising guard.

"Damion, you be good up there. Don't take any grief from anyone, and when you get out of here, come down and see me before you leave, okay, big fellow? You've been a challenge, but I kind of like you a little bit."

Damion wrote her a note saying that he was going to bring down a picture of his soccer team when he could walk again. *"Thank you for taking care of me,"* he said at the bottom of the page.

The move upstairs took about an hour because of the monitors, respirator, and other tactical concerns. Damion was welcomed back to P.I.C.U. with hugs and smiles from all the nurses. A whole new wall of cards had been hung for him, and several more balloon bouquets had come from Dothan. Neat stacks of mail lay on his bed. Everything was arranged in a warm homecoming.

More good news came. We got another no growth report from the forty-eight-hour bacteriology culture on Damion's pericardial tissue and fluid. This made everyone feel better about his antibiotic coverage and the fever that was beginning to subside.

One of the first orders of business was for Dr. Sastry to order a portable chest x-ray and to see the status of Damion's lungs before considering the removal of the two smaller side chest drains and the endotracheal tube for the respirator.

The film that came back from Radiology alarmed me. His rib cage looked like a broken bird cage that had been wired back together. His breastbone was fastened back in place with haphazard loops and twists of wire, as casually as a farmer would repair tears in a chicken coop. "Can't those sharp ends cut and irritate the tissue around them?" I asked.

No one answered. Marnix and Dr. Sastry were intent on the film's more pertinent facets like the cloudiness in the lung bases and the accompanying report from the radiologist which noted increasing underaeration at the bases, most notably on the left.

"Damion, we're not going to be able to remove your breathing tube today," Marnix told him while Terri and I finished bathing him. "But Dr. Sastry is going to order more x-rays throughout the day to see how your lungs do. If we took it out now, darling, you might struggle for air, and that would make you feel very bad again. Do you understand?"

Damion had been through this exact scenario before. He knew that his disappointment would have no impact on the time-frame of the respirator's removal. He only nodded to his dad.

"You're an angel, boy. A big patient angel," I said as I toweled off his damp and haloed hair.

The ride was becoming tumultuous again. Marnix was worried, I could see. I followed him a few moments later into our room and sat beside him on my bed as he listened on the phone and jotted notes onto his quartered and folded paper. On one side, he had written notes in preparation for his conversation with John Kelton: the usual blood values, gases, vital signs. These were followed by his worries: TTP lung relapse, breathing, nasal flare, more infiltrate in left base. All indicators were that he was heading into a flare up.

"Um huh, um huh, yes," he murmured as he quickly wrote down what John suggested. "Thanks, John. I'll get to work on these things with Sastry right away. Talk to you later.

"Anything you don't get?" Marnix asked me as he stood up to hang up the phone, aware that I had watched as he wrote.

"Do you think Sastry will let you proceed with this plasmapheresis today?" I asked, pointing to his list.

"He pretty well defers to John and me on that. I think he's taken his cue from Danny. We want every advantage we can take right now, and that means another few exchanges to taper him off."

"Despite the platelet count?"

"Despite the platelet count. That's only one indicator, the obvious one. Mary," he paused, his voice becoming more somber again, "there are other signs that the disease may be gathering strength for another attack. So we'd better be aggressive on our side."

I sighed. I felt like I couldn't stand the ups and downs another moment. Yet I had no choice. Damion had no choice.

I feel very tired today, I thought as I curled on my side for ten minutes. *I wish I could just stay in bed and sleep. My head feels cloudy, as though it too is filling up with infiltrate. And the small centers in my mind are collapsing like subsegments of his lungs in my brain's own process of atelectasis.*

"It's going to end," I murmured aloud. "At some point it is all going to end, and we will know if he lives or dies."

I rubbed my forehead to shake off this gathering dark cloud, but the haziness remained.

THURSDAY AFTERNOON

The dialysis catheter which had remained in Damion's abdomen over the last several days as a reserve system was finally removed by Dr. Swank. This didn't involve anything other than gently pulling it out and dressing the wound while Damion watched, amazed. The catheter tip was sent to the lab for culture.

Afterward, Dr. Sastry removed the two side chest tubes that weren't draining the familiar sappy pleural fluid anymore. The tips of these tubes were also sent for culture in a never ending vigilance to scan for any infection taking hold in Damion's depleted body.

Dr. Rodwig sent a nurse from the blood bank with the exchanging equipment and another supply of fresh frozen plasma to infuse. All this went off as planned so I took Marnix's advice to take a nap since Damion's spirits were raised by getting out of C.I.C.U. I gave into a numbing tiredness that was pulling me closer to the gravity of Marnix's somber attitude over these last two days. And so, for a couple of hours this afternoon, I darkened our blinds, posted a "sleeping" sign on my door, and retreated from it all.

Marnix came into the room. He sat at the foot of my bed and I listened groggily at first. "The latest x-ray is clearing," he said. "This is a huge relief. Look at the report."

He handed me the paper that by now meant everything to us. I read that Damion's lungs were clearing and there was improvement in aeration.

"Good. Maybe he can get off the respirator tomorrow. Thank you for getting him through the afternoon today. Sorry I gave out on you."

Marnix was tired now, a deeper tired than that which comes at the end of a hectic day. His weariness was what I was increasingly feeling. It was the weighty exhaustion of this having gone on for so long, through so many complications, so much sustained uncertainty about whether Damion would make it. Damion was exhausted,

I was spent, and Marnix, who'd had to balance the roles of father and doctor, who'd had to tread softly but determinedly through all the convolutions of Damion's disease, was also growing weary of the fight.

"Damion's come a long way here," I said, trying to pick him up.

But he was overcast as I was before my nap. The same darkness was bearing down on him now. "On the other hand, I want you to know Damion's got to get through who knows how many more hoops before we can take him home. He does not need pneumonia or any kind of infection. He does not need a clot. He does not need another hit on another organ. He is so beaten up now. He's so weakened that he can't afford any more major hits."

"If only we could just stop it all right now, clean up what's left, and go home. If a referee could just blow a whistle and say, 'That's it, this kid's taken enough' and call off the fight," I fantasized.

"Let's just pray we're pulling him out now. He's beyond tired. There are only so many times he can be knocked down and get up."

Marnix and I seemed to be talking this way a lot lately, as if speaking about where we were in the disease and where we needed to be going had almost become an indirect form of prayer. It was almost as if we could talk our desires into existence. We didn't have the feeling of futility that occurred at other times when we spoke this way. Somehow, we emerged from these conversations with a feeling that we were nudging our wishes closer to reality, even though we knew in more rational moments we were powerless.

"Mary, why don't you get dressed and we'll get something to eat. Then I need some sleep."

THURSDAY EVENING

As we waited for the elevator to come, the parents of the little boy whose surgery had preceded Damion's came around the corner from the direction of the pediatric rooms. They walked hand in hand and appeared to be so much more at peace, so much happier than when I last saw them in C.I.C.U.

"How's he doing?" I smiled at them.

"See for yourself," his mom beamed as Joey wheeled himself energetically along in a small wheelchair, more out of fun than necessity. He had a capped off IV line on one wrist and bore no other sign that he was a patient other than pajamas and a hospital ID bracelet.

"We're here just to finish up the IV antibiotics. Dr. Pupello thinks we can go home in a few days."

"He looks great."

As we entered the elevator, their family parade continued along the hall past the heavy doors of the pediatric intensive care unit.

THURSDAY NIGHT

While Marnix slept in our parent room and Damion slept beside me in the unit, I reflected on how Damion had survived the biggest challenge yet. The heart episode with its three taps and this last resort of stripping away the pericardium composed his biggest threat. It wasn't so much that it involved such a critical organ, or that it was coupled with pulmonary problems, or simply that it demanded the most drastic surgical intervention. The timing of his heart complications within this whole process had been so lousy. It happened when he was already malnourished, "beaten up" as Marnix described it. *Oh, thank God for getting him past all that. Thank you for letting Damion survive the roller coaster's most sickening drop yet.*

When it was this quiet in the unit I could do my best thinking. Nothing much had changed here in the last three days. A tiny infant had moved into the space that the abused child had slept in. The new baby was swaddled in gauze and connected to monitor wires and plastic respirator hoses. Even its face was muzzled by smaller versions of the ventilator tubes that Damion slept under.

"Preemie," Saracita told me. "She went home for a few days but got into lung trouble. Little, little thing." She shook her head.

Suddenly I was distracted from my reverie. The voices of Pepper and the nurses at the desk were getting louder and louder. The nurses were giggling and slapping Pepper's back as they circled around her extended left hand.

"It's true. Here's my ring to prove it!"

More laughter.

"Don't laugh! This is a two-carat ring!"

Pepper pranced in to show Sara and me. Lowering her voice so she wouldn't wake Damion, she bragged, "My doctor asked me to marry him again. This time he gave me a ring. See? Two carrots."

We looked. On her ring finger a thin strip of medical tape formed the band and held two little penciled carrots that tapered off at the knuckle. It was a cartoon ring, and we laughed too.

"Nice, huh? From scrubs to silk, here I come. This is my ticket to taking it easy the rest of my life!"

Then she spun on her white-soled shoes and swiveled her muscular hips out of the room in her exaggerated sway. It made me feel good that Pepper didn't hesitate to mock the whole married-to-a-doctor thing with me in the audience. I realized laughing that I felt more at ease with these smart tough women.

15

Another Dizzying Descent

Marnix answered the latest variation on the same question Damion had been asking for days now: when is the respirator tube coming out?

"Yes, Dr. Sastry will do it as soon as he can break away from the other side of the unit. Your chest x-ray is clearing, you're looking much better, and everyone agrees you are ready to come off it," he said.

Damion wrote his next most frequently asked question: *"Can I drink something right away?"*

"We'll have to see."

I couldn't stand this frustration for him. I superimposed a mother's empathy on a father's caution. "D., if Dr. Sastry says it's okay, I'll go out and buy a Slurpy to have ready for you when the tube comes out." I could feel Marnix's disapproval of my offer. I knew that he was worried about rushing fluids into Damion before he could adapt to drinking again. But Marnix said nothing to contradict or temper my promise. On the matter of Damion's thirst we were both parents first. We'd leave it up to the doctors to be the restrictive ones. Besides, Dr. Kiros had already been in and okayed clear fluids.

"Strawberry? Extra large?" Damion wrote.

"Strawberry. Extra large." I nodded. "If that's okay with Dr. Sastry."

"Can you ask Terri where the nearest Seven-Eleven is?"

I chuckled at his insistence. "I already have. There's a store about ten blocks away, pup. While they remove your tube, I'll drive over there and get it."

He was drawing closer and closer to his oasis. He nodded to himself and us, an earnest nod that I interpreted as, *That's good. That's good. I'm almost there.*

NOON

I cradled the big plastic container in my hands as I carefully brought it back out to my car. I'd never bought anything for my children that gratified me more. Here finally was what Damion had dreamed of and suffered over. I drove so quickly that very little had melted by the time I got back to the unit. I saw Marnix alone beside him, and Damion looking very much relieved to be free from the respirator.

"Oh, let me hear your voice!" I said.

"Hi, Mom," he said in a raspy whisper and wearing a smile. "Thanks for the drink."

His smile was all the thank you I needed. Marnix was still reluctant about giving the Slurpy to Damion but at the moment I wanted only to indulge our long-suffering son.

"Damion," Marnix said, "I know you want to guzzle this down, and I don't blame you. But start slowly, okay? Start with a couple of sips and we'll see how you do."

"Marnix, do we have to be so cautious? His NG tube is out. Kiros said he can have clear liquids. Why do we have to start so slowly?"

"Just do it my way, okay?" he said to us both. "It's been a long time since Damion's G.I. tract has been challenged. Damion, you might get nauseated if you start too quickly. And I don't understand why we have to start with something frozen," Marnix said disapprovingly to me.

"Because, out of everything he's dreamed of drinking, this is what he wanted the most. Look, let's not fuss about this. Marnix, you compromise by letting him have his favorite drink. D., you compromise by having just a little to begin with. The rest can go in the nurses' freezer. That's fair, isn't it?"

Marnix looked on reluctantly as Damion unwrapped the plastic straw and punctured the cross slit in the cover. He raised the Slurpy almost ceremoniously to his lips and drew in two large mouthfuls, pausing to swallow in between. He handed the drink to me and I took it to the freezer in the nurses' lounge behind the central desk.

"Happy to drink, is he?" As I was passing, Dr. Sastry looked up from his paperwork.

"Very happy. And to be off the ventilator and to have the NG tube out of his nose. Thanks for all that this morning."

"He's doing very well, very much better today," Dr. Sastry said in his rapid fire Indian accent.

Except for his lungs, Damion's problems seemed to be resolving, and it seemed logical they would improve as soon as he could sit upright. Marnix and I sat with Damion over the next few minutes, talking quietly about how long it might take before he could get onto the regular floor, and beyond that how long it might be before he could be discharged from the hospital altogether.

Suddenly Damion blanched, curled over onto his side, and winced as he fumbled for his pain pump. Before we could react, he pushed in the plunger four times, unloading a strong dose of morphine into his IV. This was the first time he had given himself pain medication since the early hours in the recovery room.

"What's the matter, D.?"

"What is it, baby?"

"It hurts."

"Show me where."

Damion pointed to his lower abdomen, but wouldn't uncurl from the fetal position. Marnix leaned over and stroked Damion's hair until he dozed off from the morphine. Then he settled deep back in his armchair and stared severely at Damion.

"What was that?" I asked.

"That," Marnix glared in a very measured and distinctly angry pronunciation, "was a perforation."

"What?" I asked disbelieving.

"Our son has just blown a hole in his bowel."

"Come on, Marnix, please don't say that."

It can't possibly be, I thought to myself. Damion's just cramping. He's just unaccustomed to drinking or eating. Marnix is reading too much into it.

Marnix sat very quietly, watching Damion and the monitor numbers. Then be slowly rose and went out of the room to talk to

Sastry at the desk. In a few moments they came back in together. Dr. Sastry watched Damion, touched his skin, and studied the monitor. He left and found Terri who had been in and out all morning, but who had been away during this last half hour. They talked quietly at the large desk. Marnix settled back in his chair, propped his brow on two fingers, and watched.

"What does Sastry think of your concern?"

"He thinks I am overreacting."

"Marnix, it should be okay. Look how everything is stable, all his numbers are good. I think he's just got pain from having to learn to handle fluids all over again."

"You don't understand. It won't be immediate. But wait, just wait."

I shifted in the nearby chair, praying for the best, fearing the worst.

Over the next two hours we watched Damion sleep a drugged sleep. Everything stayed the same on his monitor, other than a slight elevation in his heart rate and blood pressure. Marnix started writing notes on a clean sheet of quartered paper. By now I knew how and why he did this. His formula was to sort out three categories about the case: his instincts, the actual information, and possible directions.

I felt very guilty about the drink I'd bought Damion and being part of the cause for Marnix's stress as he rose one more time to walk toward Dr. Sastry. It was nearly three o'clock. They talked a long while and eventually left together. In ten more minutes Dr. Sastry reentered the unit with Terri, who came over to Damion's space and asked me to follow her. She led me through different P.I.C.U. doors that opened up to a less traveled corridor.

"Terri, do you know where Marnix went?"

"I think he's in your parent room. Listen, I've got to talk to you."

She stumbled for the words to say what she had to diplomatically. "This has been very hard on you both. On all of us. It's a prolonged disease, and Damion's been through a lot over the last three weeks. His dad has been absolutely great, but . . ."

"But what?"

"He needs to stop imagining the worst. Like right now, about a little abdominal pain from drinking."

"Terri, I was there. That was not a little pain. Damion had a terrible reaction a few minutes after drinking."

A strand of hair had fallen over her eyes. "But it's normal that after cardiac surgery he would still be in pain."

"This wasn't in his chest. It was abdominal."

She smoothed her hair back from her face. "What I'm saying is this is very hard for any parent. And you guys have been great. Parents are an essential part of the team for kids up here. It's even harder for any parent with a medical background because they know too much. They know what can go wrong. Your husband's stressed out and tired from the whole thing. Will you talk to him for us?"

I shook my head. "No, because I'm not sure Marnix is wrong. I presume Dr. Sastry has expressed this to him directly?"

"I'm not sure. I didn't hear them speak."

"Well, come on with me. You know that Marnix has a high regard for you. We both do. You've been incredibly devoted to Damion from day one. You talk to him if you're absolutely convinced Damion's okay."

I led her to our room and asked Marnix to come and talk to her as soon as he got off the phone. Terri and I waited quietly in the hall until he came out a few moments later.

"Marnix, Terri has some concerns about us being very worn out. And specifically about how you may be overly worried because not only are you a parent but your medical background makes you see all the things that can go badly. Is that essentially it, Terri?" I asked her.

Terri breathed in deeply. While she thought about how to talk to him, I excused myself and went back to the unit using the doors that kept me from passing Dr. Sastry.

"What did Sastry have to say to you?" I asked him.

"About the same thing Terri had to say."

"Marnix." I took a deep breath. "I don't agree with them. I'm hoping you're wrong and they're right about this, but I do respect your judgment. The good thing is that his numbers still look good, and he's sleeping well."

"He's sleeping well because he's knocked out with morphine."

"But don't you think he *could* be okay and that reaction was maybe a blip of some sort?"

"No, I know I'm right on this. He has a perforated intestine."

"Well, is there something we can ask for—an x-ray or an ultrasound or something?"

"No. It's shift change time around here. Everyone's in the middle of going home. Closing up shop for the weekend," he said with frustration but without any true cynicism in his voice.

"Are you saying that has anything to do with them not taking you seriously on this?"

"All I can say is that it's Friday afternoon at 4:10. Sastry's leaving now. Nurses are switching over. I am accused of being the tired one, when they can't wait to wrap up the week and get out of here. I'm being admonished to play by the rules, so that's what we'll do. We'll sit here and wait for what's coming and hope we didn't waste too much time once we all see the shit hit the fan."

I felt crestfallen. Another sharp descent for Damion to endure.

I leaned over and, careful not to wake him, I put my hand on Damion's side, then his forehead and cried out, "Holy Christ! He's burning up!"

Marnix jumped up and grabbed a digital thermometer off the supply tray, ripped off its sleeve, and placed its tip under Damion's tongue. Damion stirred groggily, but didn't awaken. We watched the numbers steadily climb. Finally, it beeped at 104.1.

"Oh my God!" Marnix said plaintively as he sat back down to try and figure out what his next move should be. The central desk was empty.

"Marnix, I'm so sorry about the drink."

"Mary, dear, it's not your fault. It would have happened whatever he drank. Who should I call?" he asked himself.

"If this is an acute belly," I offered, "then I assume we need help right away. Don't you think Kiros can line up the right people?"

"Good idea. That's it. I'll call Kiros. He can start channeling everything and will be one less link in the chain of command to go over."

Marnix snatched up his papers and darted out the unit doors to our room. I fingered the silver-tipped thermometer with 104.1 now frozen in its liquid crystal window.

"I can't believe this!" I murmured. This was where we had started, with gastroenterology and Kiros. I didn't remember anything in Dr. Havis's roller coaster metaphor that suggested once you made it around the entire track, you had to repeat the same dizzying course all over again.

FRIDAY EVENING AND NIGHT

In a hospital, time can be slowed to a state of ennui. Large chunks of Damion's eighteen days had gone that way, time dissolving into a long chain of tedium.

But, during a crisis, time assumed an alarmingly high velocity consistent with the roller coaster analogy of Damion's disease. At times of plummeting danger when Damion had fallen into more complications, time had careened wildly out of control. Then all we could feel was a sickening acceleration and a nauseating descent into the next peril. After he bottomed out, time would slow again. Now, time began its free fall again. From 4:15 on, time, events, and people flew by in a world streaked with danger.

Marnix called Dr. Kiros. "I feel funny calling you on my own but I feel you have the best expertise on his belly." And Marnix went on to describe Damion's symptoms.

Then, Dr. Kiros came in and checked Damion. But because Damion was still sleepy from the morphine and his temperature had dropped a little, Dr. Kiros felt he was doing reasonably well. He explained to us, "Damion's intestinal tract had essentially shut down for three weeks. It can be a painful and slow process for the body to relearn how to handle fluids and food again." He paused. "The fever's not surprising in light of how it had hovered around a hundred and two ever since the pericardial tap on Tuesday. Remember, this fever has abated only one day over the last four, and his temperature was likely to be inconsistent for a while."

In all Dr. Kiros was very kind, gave us lots of time, but came to the same conclusion the others had, that nothing drastic was going on.

Marnix and I sat in stunned silence when he left. Damion flitted in and out of sleep, never asking for anything to drink when he awoke. He seemed listless and disconnected again as he emerged slowly from the drugged afternoon. We checked his temperature frequently and watched it steadily begin to elevate again. Marnix was more or less dumbfounded about what to do next.

"I'm sure about this. I'm positive," he said in between Damion's waking spells and Saracita's entrances and exits.

"I know he's in trouble," he repeated.

"Marnix, you haven't eaten anything all day. Why don't you go down and grab a quick bite. I'll stay by him."

"All right. What do you want? I'll bring it up and you can eat it in our room."

"Nothing right now."

As Marnix rose to leave our space, Dr. Swank came into the unit and walked toward us. Marnix jumped at this last chance to communicate his instincts about Damion's condition to someone. He caught him at the door. They spoke quickly and quietly, and then came in together.

Dr. Swank nodded to me and immediately lifted the corner of the sheet over the peritoneal dialysis dressing. Dr. Swank usually only came to see Damion when surgical matters arose or for follow-up work. We had seen him most recently yesterday when he had come to remove the dialysis catheter. When he touched Damion's skin, his left eyebrow rose.

"He's quite hot."

"It was one-o-four point one earlier," Marnix volunteered. "It's climbing back up now."

"Has he been sleeping like this all afternoon?"

"Ever since he gave himself the maximum dosage of morphine."

Dr. Swank woke Damion and palpated his belly, starting right below the dressing covering his chest incision and working his way down the sides of his swollen abdomen. Damion became increasingly uncomfortable with every inch Dr. Swank's hands advanced, until finally Damion cried out and tried to guard his lower left side.

"Sorry, Damion," Dr. Swank said.

"He is distended. You're correct about the guarding and the

temperature. Let's get a portable x-ray of his abdomen. I've got surgery in a few minutes. I'll call Radiology, and get them to call in the findings to me."

Dr. Swank looked at his watch. "I'll be back to check on you, Damion. Nothing to drink or eat, and no pain medications until I do. Understand?"

Soon the massive portable x-ray machine announced itself. It rolled along with a primitive rumble that we recognized as soon as it was unloaded from the service elevator far away. By now Damion was in so much pain that positioning him properly for the angles that Dr. Swank had ordered was very difficult. Marnix wore one of the lead aprons as he propped Damion up for a side view by rolling him on his side and holding him and the x-ray cassettes in place so the technician could expose the films.

"Sorry, man. I know it hurts, but let's get one more side view while your dad holds you still."

When Dr. Swank came back to the unit we spoke with him between Damion's cubicle and the unmanned desk. "The film showed free air in the abdomen. The small bowel loops show evidence of distention," he said looking at Marnix.

"He's got an acute abdomen," Dr. Swank said to me. "The only way to get free air into the peritoneal space like this would be through an intestinal perforation." He continued for both of us, "We need to do an emergency exploratory tonight, as soon as I can free up an O.R."

"Is he going to be put back on the ventilator?" I asked weakly. "Yes."

"Damion's going to have a hard time with that. He just got off it again," I said sadly.

"We're looking at an involved procedure here with a general anesthesia. We're going to have to cut from his sternotomy incision down to his pelvic region to give me enough room to dissect his G.I. tract and repair whatever's responsible. His general condition is already compromised and I don't know what I'll find once I get in. So what are you getting at with this concern over the ventilator?" he asked me severely.

"I'm asking you that if he must be intubated only for the surgery, and it's likely that in recovery he'll be extubated before he comes to, can we all give him a break, and not even tell him about the respirator?"

Dr. Swank looked at me skeptically. I hadn't explained this very well. I tried again. "I sense that it's really getting to be a problem for Damion, to the point where I worry he's going to say to himself going into this surgery, 'It's not worth it anymore.' I think it might affect how hard he fights. That's all I'm asking. Please don't tell him if you don't have to."

Dr. Swank did not budge. He looked so much like my father. He dressed like him, and he had the same stern midwestern manner, tall physique, prematurely gray hair and good looks. He also had the same no-nonsense, straight-shooting approach.

"Mrs. Heersink, I am not going to lie to your son for you," he said, an edge of steel in his voice.

And then he turned abruptly to tell Damion about the surgery he'd have that night. We listened in at the door. Damion's one and only question to Dr. Swank was a quivering, "Do I have to be back on the respirator?"

"See what I mean?" I mouthed to Marnix.

Then I left to go to our parent room. I left the doctors to answer that one for Damion.

Marnix soon joined me in our room.

"It wasn't a lot to ask," I defended. "To downplay the respirator thing if he could. I don't think Damion can take too much more of it."

"Mary, you've got to see Swank's point. He comes in here Friday evening on a simple errand like rounds and finds this complicated mess on his hands. He doesn't know when he's going to be able to squeeze Damion in between all the trauma that the ER keeps sending up to the OR on Friday nights when the city goes wild. He's worried over what he'll find when he opens D. up. And now this mother starts asking him not to be straightforward with this bright, inquisitive child. He's not going to do that for you, nor should he."

"Look, Dr. Swank has no idea what I was trying to say. I wasn't asking to keep Damion off the respirator. I just wanted to please spare him the anxiety by not telling him."

"That's unrealistic. You heard Damion's first question."

"Yeah, and I'd really like to know how sensitively it was answered. No one appreciates what the respirator means to our son like I do. I'm very worried it will keep Damion from trying. That is how sick he is of it."

Marnix didn't answer. This was the kind of conflict that was impossible to choose sides on. Both Dr. Swank's honesty and my worry were correct. However, to tell or not to tell Damion was not the most critical issue at the moment.

"I'm sorry, Marnix. I know it was an inappropriate thing to ask in the scheme of things. It was stupid to even bring it up. It's just that this whole thing stinks more and more. Our kid never gets a break. Every time he survives the struggles back up the incline, he finds out he has to go down to the bottom again. It just can't keep going like this. Forget the respirator. Sorry I ever mentioned it, especially to Damion's most aloof doctor."

"You shouldn't say that. He's good, Mary, very good. Not to mention he saved D. by coming in tonight," Marnix corrected me.

Marnix was right, and I knew it but there were more critical things here. "What are we in for here? Can you honestly tell me how bad this one is?" I asked.

Marnix's voice was grave. "People with perforated bowels survive all the time if they're repaired in time. But Damion's very weakened now. And the infection just gets nastier as time goes on. He does not need this bacterial spillage fomenting in him all night. There's no doubt that Swank's visit was a godsend."

I nodded. I had been unfair to Dr. Swank.

"You know one thing I don't understand? Why now? If his colon was going to blow, why didn't it perforate early on in the disease when it was even more ravaged? Why are we coming back to where we started?"

"No one can be sure, especially till we see what's going on inside. It could be a weakened area, or an area that's been dead all this time but because we weren't challenging his G.I. tract with fluids and food, it managed to hold together. Or this could be a clot that's hit the intestine and is killing off a section there now. That's why I've been so insistent on not rushing to end plasmapheresis."

"Kind of ironic, isn't it? Don't you find it strange that we've come full circle, back to a gastrointestinal complication?"

Marnix shook his head. "No one can predict what organ this disease will hit next."

It helped us to speak theoretically. We should have kept our discussion of a perforation on that conceptual level. The fact that we didn't threw me into the deepest abyss, cut me to the core, and made something happen that we'd managed to avoid throughout the entire process of getting through this disease as a couple. Here was where we violated for the first time our essential rule of self-defense, if only momentarily. Our conversation made everything inside me crumble, and worse, broke our golden rule of never thinking at the same time that Damion would die.

I started it by asking, "How's Dr. Swank going to do this? I mean, what's the surgery going to look like?"

Marnix was brutally honest.

"He's going to have to lift everything out as best he can and go through Damion's intestines inch by inch looking for ruptures. He's got to suture the ruptures, wash everything down and then repack the organs as best he can in the peritoneal space."

"Are you serious? He's got to take everything out?"

This was horrible! I should have stopped there. This was more than enough to throw me into despair. I should never have asked him the next question. "What do you think he'll find when he gets in?"

Marnix's answer was curt. "He could find something simple. Or Damion may end up losing three-quarters of his colon. But another possibility when he opens Damion up is that he could see that his intestines are so shredded and dissolved that . . ."

He paused and looked away from me, perhaps knowing how dangerous it was to complete his thought.

"That what?" I pressed.

He sighed. "That it would be impossible to fix that much damage."

"Oh." My despair careened to bottom. "You mean that's a possibility? And how likely is that?"

He still kept his eyes averted from me. "I don't know. But it's one to consider."

"Oh." My words trailed off.

After a few minutes of neither of us saying a word, I stood up and touched him on the shoulder.

"I need to sit with Damion until they take him down."

"I'll be there in a little while," Marnix said softly.

I understood his heartbreak and he understood mine. He needed to be alone. I needed to be with Damion.

It was after 10:00. Sara sat by Damion who was in great discomfort by now. She kept cool rags on his forehead, and spoke to him softly and encouraged him that the surgery would fix the pain in his belly. She had given him what medication Dr. Swank had ordered, but it wasn't putting a dent in his agony.

"It won't be long, darling, before they take you down," I said, bending to kiss Damion's burning cheek.

Sara had turned off the lights at Damion's request. So the three of us sat in the muted light that entered through the tilted blinds. I was glad at least that Damion and Sara could not see me cry.

But Sara did feel my agony. As time passed and Damion drifted off to a light sleep, she stood up and whispered in my ear, "Hang in there, darling. He's going to make it."

"I don't know, Sara. He's come all this way in all these weeks. He's not even over his cardiac surgery, and now this. I think time's running out. There's no way he can keep this up forever."

Sara patted my back. Her kindness to me made even more tears come. She handed me a box of tissues and sat back down. The rest of the night, as Marnix came in and out, she looked at me almost as often as she watched over Damion. Time inched by.

Sara's shift ended but she stayed on and sat with us. The next nurse was Denita, a relatively new face for us, and very nice, too. But having Sara wait with us made me feel better. She was stoic yet optimistic. I was glad she was there.

It was after 11:00 before a phone call at the desk informed the nurses that the orderlies would be up to get Damion.

"I'll come down with you," Sara volunteered when the orderlies had gotten Damion and his equipment transferred to the gurney. Denita came with us, too. Marnix and I, Sara, Denita, and two orderlies all formed a tight procession around the gurney and crammed into the patient elevator.

Damion was was in a lot of pain. He was nervous. I wanted it all to be over and yet I wanted the elevator ride to take forever. I didn't want to surrender him to the paper clothed nurses again at the entrance to the operating room. But it all happened so fast, like the pushing of the button on the roller coaster ride which accelerates the process. There wasn't time to say goodbye this time. When they wheeled him in and his hands slipped out of ours, there was no reason to hold back my tears any longer. I walked away from the group and found a darkened lounge to sit alone in. Marnix stayed behind with Sara and Denita and talked to them in a serious hunched-over manner. I was talked out.

Why didn't he just let them go back up to the unit and come sit with me? I wondered.

Moments later all three of them walked into the waiting area. They looked worried. I did not even try to say something uplifting. I could not stop crying. My own emotions had careened out of control.

"Mary, I want Denita to stay with us. Sara has to go home now. She was good to stay over for us this long."

"Thank you very much, but I don't want you to stay, Denita. I'll be all right." I sobbed brokenly. "I just need to be alone with Marnix for a while. Look, you all don't have to be worried about me. I'm sorry I can't stop crying, but I'll be okay."

They didn't do what I asked. Instead, they propelled me towards the cafeteria, the last place on earth I wanted to be. They talked like everything was going to work out, and fussed over getting me something to eat and drink as if this was the most important thing anyone could do.

"You all are very nice to worry about it but I don't want anything," I protested in vain. Fortunately the cafeteria was nearly empty. Not many people would see me crying here. I hated to be emotional in front of people. Marnix and Denita pulled me along the food line as they pointed out yogurt, cookies, and fruit. They seemed to be implying if I'd just eat something, everything would somehow be better, as if my blood sugar level was the underlying cause of this colossal disaster.

Why was this uncontrollable grief happening? It was something that I lost that night. Something that I had to surrender. And I knew even if Damion would be granted a reprieve, what I lost would never be returned to me. What I lost was the sense of trust that I needed to live happily, blissfully. It was a faith in the beautiful collective myths and dreamy lies that made life manageable. It was like glimpsing something inherently evil that we are not supposed to see.

Standing sobbing in front of the salads and glazed donuts, I thought about everything we'd endured over the past month. When I drove Damion to the emergency room, I had sensed evil. *But I still believed in everything.* I believed all the lies that many in the world harbor still. I believed in the creed of medicine and that antibiotics could defeat any bug. I believed that children in a developed country at the end of the twentieth century could not get sick and die from contamination in federally inspected food. I believed in the wholesomeness implicit in the USDA seal of approval stamped on all the meat sold in this country. I believed in these dangerous myths that lulled us all into complacency. I believed in the even more basic lie that was harder to surrender: our inalienable right to happiness. Until slowly, wrenchingly, through crisis after crisis, I saw promises I'd once tightly held ripped away as this mysterious bacterium did its damage. I saw Damion plummeting, climbing back up, falling down again. I saw complications and crash after crash while he struggled to stay alive.

Some people come to a place after which nothing will be the same in their lives again, a defining place that changes their path for the rest of their lives. For me it occurred unexpectedly there in that deserted hospital cafeteria. That's when something inside me was severed. The final and most beautiful illusion of all was cut from me. It was when I had to relinquish the biggest lie that every parent cherishes: *the lie that our children belong to us.* It was the lie that Damion was mine and that somehow people would keep rescuing him and that we could keep him and all would be well.

It was after midnight. I was standing in front of a wide-eyed, middle-aged black woman who looked at me in bewilderment from behind the cash register. She didn't know what to do about me. Marnix was confused, too. He just wanted me to pay for the carton of milk and walk over to a table with Denita tagging along. Through everything before, even the cardiac surgery, I had been reasonably composed and even useful to him. Now I was unraveling, weeping miserably, unable to stop.

And Damion was in the operating room again with everyone expecting the worst, his body opened up again. His swollen intestines were being lifted out of his body cavity and mounded onto his draped chest. Dr. Swank was unwinding them inch by steaming inch, looking for rips. After repairs, all would have to be hosed down with the strongest antibiotics, and the cavity washed out before being repacked with the organs. And here was I in a cafeteria, with everyone wanting me to buy this milk. I could not. I was crying and crying and crying. It was then I realized that I had to get ready for my child to die soon. *And this could be the time.*

I had to give up everything to let him die. So that was what I did, as I paid for the milk. Then I swore bitterly to Marnix, the nurse, and the amazed cashier, "I will never, never, ever believe in anything false again! In fact," the crying now finished, "I will not believe in anything again."

16

A Kind of Darkness

MARNIX AND I sat on a small couch. I curled up beside him and put my head on his lap. Finally, I said, "Marnix, I understand now what our fight was about, why you were angry with me. I really did think I could demand a cure, and Damion would make it. You were right that I thought we could make him live. How on earth did I ever get that stupid idea, acting like a spoiled child?"

"Hush," he whispered.

Just then Dr. Swank appeared in his scrubs, his paper hat still on his head. We jumped up and stared at him.

"Well, it's done. Damion's in the Recovery Room in satisfactory condition. He came through it just fine."

That's what we needed to hear. That's what we longed to hear, Dr. Swank. That's what will make us soar again. But despite the news I was still numb.

"It's quite surprising what I found," Dr. Swank said. "The small bowel appeared to be normal but I noticed a hematoma at the ligament of Treitz. I took down the ligament but still couldn't find a reason for the hematoma."

Dr. Swank seemed to be setting up the background for what he found so unique: "As I mobilized his left upper quadrant I found fecal matter on the transverse colon, right at the splenic flexure. I brought this over and cleaned it off. Now this is what is surprising. I found a discrete perforation about seven millimeters in diameter. It looked just like a bullet hole."

"A bullet hole?"

"Not the kind of thing you ever see in kids. An ischemic looking hole.

"Anyway, I got good closure on the hole and we rinsed out the abdominal cavity with Neosporin. I didn't find any other perforations. I replaced the bowel and sutured him back up. All in all he did well. His blood loss was probably no more than fifty milliliters."

Dr. Swank looked exhausted. I thought about how hard it would be to perform surgery for eighteen hours straight.

"You can go into Recovery and see him now," he said. Then he remembered something and turned toward me. "He'll be better off tonight on the respirator. Tomorrow the P.I.C.U. can make a determination what to do based on his pulmonary picture."

Marnix expressed our thanks while I stood back more or less dead inside, listening to what this surgeon had found and thinking that Damion had made another narrow escape.

"Dr. Swank, thank you for coming in tonight. Thank you for what you've done. We can never thank you enough for tonight," Marnix was saying.

After he left, we stood alone a minute before going to Damion.

At the same time we both said, "A bullet hole? Shaped like a bullet hole?"

"Thank God for intestinal perforations that are as neat and precise as bullet holes," Marnix said as he hugged me.

I was still rooted to the spot, grateful for the news that made Marnix ecstatic, grateful that Damion was still here, but insensate from the devastating lesson I had finally learned this night.

LATE SATURDAY MORNING

Damion slept through most of the morning, presumably because of the anesthesia slowly wearing off. This seemed merciful to me. Every hour he slept was one less he had to be hostage to the respirator. He would not get the tube out today: the early morning chest x-ray showed fluid infiltrating in his lower left lobe, the most stubborn part of his lungs to clear. It was slightly worse than yesterday's picture.

When Dr. Sastry came into the unit, nothing was said about the day before. Better to focus on where we were now rather than allow past events to ferment into what could only hurt Damion in the long run.

John Kelton made several suggestions to guard against post-operative complications. All of them were immediately embraced by Dr. Sastry and implemented.

Today two doses of heparin were pumped into Damion's IV. The infarct to his intestine was evidence enough to Dr. Swank that the anticoagulant would be in order. And Damion's platelet count had climbed into the low range of normal, so fears of hemorrhage were lessened.

Even with the heparin, Marnix and John remained worried about recurrence of another clot like the one that made the hole in Damion's colon. Yesterday's perforation was a clear sign that the disease had not run its course. They lobbied for more plasmapheresis. Again, Dr. Sastry deferred.

Whenever Damion woke up, the severe pain he'd experienced the day before seemed abated. Marnix insisted the morphine pump be removed because morphine, as we saw the day before, could mask the symptoms of another bowel perforation. Damion remained quiet, groggy, and sometimes confused throughout the day.

Finally, Dr. Swank called in the same specialist who had given Damion a cursory glance during our first days at St. Joseph's. While he flipped through Damion's thick chart, I watched him, my anger crystallizing. Had he read the articles, I wondered. Was he unaware of E. coli 0157:H7, this new, incendiary pathogen and its relevance to our son's disease? Had he read the articles coming out attributing H.U.S. cases to the killer microbe?

I could have asked him about it, I supposed, but we needed him badly to keep Damion from major infection. As I bit my lip, I wondered if I had now started playing by the rules of what Marnix described as the politics of medicine?

What happened, doctor? I thought to myself as he spent five minutes with Damion this morning.

By the time the specialist left, I had convinced myself that it was best to give this man the benefit of the doubt. I imagined a whole generation of clinicians who must be playing catch up with a mysterious bacterium, which now, years past their medical training, had burst virulently on the scene. But wasn't it weird? *How could this material come circuitously to us, how could it be right around the corner in our bureau when it missed him entirely, he whose job it was to keep up with emerging infectious agents?*

It was a day of lining up the weaponry Damion needed if the battle wasn't over. Damion did pretty well, Marnix rallied, and I just watched, more or less amazed our son was still alive.

SATURDAY EVENING

"D.D., do you want to watch the Duke-Iowa game with me?" Marnix asked. "Dr. Kelton told me he needs you to cheer for Duke. This'll be the second round of the NCAA tournament. If they win this, they can go on to Philadelphia Wednesday night, and maybe even win a national championship a second year in a row."

The blue light of the television infused Marnix's and Damion's faces with radiance. For a moment they could have been back in our bedroom at home watching sports. "See the little guy, number 11? That's Bobby Hurley. He's someone who won't give up. Can you believe that he broke his foot in February and kept playing that game anyway? Almost everyone thought he was finished for the season, but now he's back to being a team leader. Look at that! Look how he gets in there every time. Nice!!"

This was their territory. I left them when half-time was coming up, with Duke ahead 48-24. Marnix leaned all the way back in the armchair under the monitor screen with his feet propped on the bottom rail of Damion's bed. Damion's face was fixed on the television overhead. Despite the respirator and the incision that ran all the way up his torso, the chest tubes and the machines, the image of the two of them recaptured the normalcy their lives had before: the sweetness of a dad and a boy watching a game.

"Whoa! What a shot! You're going to fire off three pointers like that someday."

D's eyes squinted in happiness.

SUNDAY MORNING, MARCH 22

Damion was quiet and stable. His heart rate had dropped to 135, his blood pressure was 140 over 95, and his temperature was only slightly above normal. His blood gases looked good, his chemistries better. An x-ray study of his abdomen showed a slightly greater than usual amount of gas in the colon, but an amount within normal limits. Marnix heard bowel sounds when he borrowed the nurse's stethoscope. Most indicators showed that Damion was pulling out of this latest assault as well as could be hoped for.

The overriding concern was infection. It overshadowed even the cardiopulmonary concerns of the last two weeks, despite today's unchanged heart enlargement and pulmonary infiltrate.

We were taking a break in our room. "Marnix. Do you ever think about the number of ironies we bump into throughout this whole process? They just amaze me. Think about the latest. We start with an infection. Here we are weeks later trying our best to avoid an infection."

Marnix listened without comment.

I took a deep breath. "And another irony, a deeper one. The disease was set in motion by fecal contamination when a cow's gut was split during slaughter. And here we are a month later, a whole chain reaction of disease later and Damion ends up infecting his own sterile tissue when fecal contamination spills out of *his* bowel."

I followed Marnix as he walked toward our dresser. There was a chance he might go home tonight for a few days if Damion did well all day. He had to make some tentative flight reservations.

"It's sort of the whole mechanism in microcosm. And kind of evil, too, in the way it all ends up a circle."

Marnix remained focused on the task at hand, sorting through the airline folders for flight times to Tallahassee. I didn't know if he was even listening to my musings. But I was sure I was right. It was all a circle. What started out as fecal contamination in the slaughterhouse had come to rounded fruition when spillage of Damion's own intestinal contents threatened his life again.

Damion's favorite respiratory therapist, a young black man named Robert with an easy laid back manner, was giving him his treatment. Robert chatted with him about the game last night as if he were conducting a two-way conversation when suddenly Damion coughed and dislodged the endotracheal tube which aided his breathing.

We all stared at it, surprised.

The foot-long, mucus-covered tube lay on his chest. "Sorry, I didn't mean it," Damion said sheepishly.

"I can't believe this," Robert said. "How did you do that, Damion? You just coughed it out."

Dr. Sastry was unavailable, busy on the other side of the unit. So we all waited and watched the oxygenation numbers and Damion's respiration, which stayed in the reasonable range of twenty a minute. Within a half hour, Dr. Sastry came over and saw what had happened. There was a discussion of what to do, the end result of which was to do nothing other than watch him. "If he can manage without the respirator, I won't intubate him again," Dr. Sastry announced.

"Well, I guess when you said you wanted it out you meant business," Robert said as he packed up his bag. "I don't see too many patients take matters into their own hands. Spitting their own tube out. You are just too much," he laughed.

SUNDAY AFTERNOON

Parents living in a hospital inevitably pick up its unique language. Certain situations, too graphic to spell out for visitors, are discreetly referred to in code. The most frightening signal at St. Joseph's, one that families soon learned to dread, was Code 19. It was the death code.

We were downstairs in the cafeteria trying to get a half-hour distraction when over the loud speaker system the fearful code was announced. "P.I.C.U., Code nineteen. P.I.C.U., Code nineteen." We heard it and flinched.

Marnix and I sat not too far from the only parental faces we recognized. Boo Man's mother and father were becoming bleak fixtures in our world. They were still here hanging onto the hope that someday he'd wake up. Although his basic physical functions had stabilized over the last weeks, he showed no neurological progress. When I relayed updates to Marnix, he'd just shake his head as if to say, no way. Beyond that, Marnix's nonresponse told me how uncomfortable he was in hearing about other children's cases at this point. He wanted to protect himself. His own child's struggle was more than enough to deal with.

When the Code 19 sounded, Boo Man's parents stared at us, and we stared back. Three of the nurses from the pediatric floor and two men in scrubs jumped up at once and rushed out leaving their unfinished food behind. Boo's parents left also, depositing their trays on the conveyor belt near the exit.

"It's not us. It can't be," I said, trying to disguise my concern.

"No. He's doing too well. We're okay."

I reviewed the children I knew on our side of the pediatric intensive care unit. It wasn't Marty. There was the little preemie all wrapped in gauze under the respirator. There was a new two-year-old who had come the night before with an intestinal problem. It could be him: his red-faced parents seemed very distraught. Other than Boo Man, I didn't know any children on the other side of the unit. With its own separate facilities, that side of P.I.C.U. might as well be ten miles away.

"Damion is doing much better today," I repeated to reassure Marnix and me.

Marnix concurred. "He is. If this were any of the shakier times, we'd be flying up there right now."

"But he's okay. Thank God, he's okay today," I emphasized.

In five minutes, not sooner so that we didn't allow ourselves the slightest impression that this Code 19 could be related to us, Marnix and I walked at a deliberately normal pace toward the elevators. When we got to the eighth floor, we found Boo Man's parents and the parents of the new toddler locked out of two sets of swinging doors. No one could get in or out until this crisis was resolved. The toddler on our side must be all right because his parents didn't seem upset. Boo Man's parents were just very quiet. They leaned against the wall on their side of the hall, looking downward.

Soon the doors to the other side of the unit parted. For an instant we saw the dark clothes of the men dispatched whenever a patient "codes." They were leaning on the desk talking to a group of nurses. A nurse came through the doors and saw us. She went over to Boo Man's mom and dad, touching their arms reassuringly.

"It's not him. You know that, don't you?"

They continued looking down and nodded yes. I knew what they were feeling. Even if it were not the child of any one of us, we all felt that it could have been ours.

"It's all right," the nurse answered a question that none of us asked, but all of us had thought. "It worked out. You can all go in now."

She opened the door for Boo Man's parents to enter, then lifted the wall phone and instructed our desk nurse to unlock our unit. We followed the anxious new couple. As we continued past their cubicle, I saw that their child was a beautiful baby with a sweet round face and golden hair in a bowl cut like our Bayne's. But this child looked terribly sick, as pitifully beautiful as a broken cherub.

SUNDAY NIGHT

As we drove to the airport for Marnix to catch his flight, we were plunged again into the strangeness of the real world outside the hospital walls. Everything looked so extreme. Lights blazed in the deserted stadium parking lot. Illuminated fountains in front of office buildings shimmered and caught the eye of those in passing traffic. Sleek corporate headquarters pierced the flat land, skyward temples to an earlier prosperity. Now their empty offices were excessively lit and their grounds were landscaped as intemperately as an amusement park. All of this took control of our senses and our weary minds as we drove along the streets.

"Hey, don't you think Tampa looks better at night?" I said.

Marnix didn't respond. He was thinking of something else.

"I'm glad your sister is arriving tomorrow," he said pensively. "Grace's nurse's perspective is valuable. I feel better about leaving knowing she'll be here, especially in light of John's advice about the stage he thinks we're entering."

"I know."

"She'll see things we can't," he said confidently. "And you'll review with her the things we have to watch?"

He meant all the charts, signs, and indicators he had written out in long lists for me to record and call in to him throughout the day. It was hard for him to leave, but the other children and his practice demanded it. Over the last three weeks, he'd only managed to see patients two-thirds of one day, and that was the day he'd had to turn around and come back for the heart surgery. His staff was rescheduling patients, clearing the books, and delaying surgeries the best they could. But eventually the backlog would become critical. Marnix never mentioned the office but I could imagine the mess.

Marnix's plan was to squeeze in two, maybe three, days and then fly back. This appeared to be good timing. Damion's spirits were level. Danny was coming in tomorrow for the week.

"The key thing," Marnix said, "is the danger of becoming tired. We're all falling prey to exhaustion: Damion, the doctors, the nurses, you and me. Everyone is emotionally drained and fed up with the disease. John says this is typical. H.U.S. lasts so long that it becomes a marathon for the doctors and nurses. Now is the point where people slip. We saw that Friday with the perforation. People get tired and begin to miss symptoms. Little things turn into big things. Now when everyone is most depleted is the time for greater attention to detail and emphasis on meticulous care. Watch the sterile technique. Change lines and dressings frequently. Watch the meds and nutrition. Watch everything like a hawk!

"The nurses have to be our greatest allies in this phase. John says continue to show them our gratitude. Don't take them for granted. They're the ones who must carry out the care he needs. And they're emotionally tired of this case now. This is when tempers get frayed and misunderstandings flare."

"Like what happened with Terri on Friday afternoon."

"Exactly. John tells me it's amazing the number of kids that get through the most catastrophic events only to stumble on a technicality at the end. 'Don't lose Damion on a technicality,' he always warns me.

"Meticulous care, meticulous care," Marnix repeated like a mantra, emphasizing for me the current guiding principle. "That's why it's good that Grace is coming. She'll come in fresh and will notice the details."

I pulled into a gap in the line of cars unloading passengers.

"Well, we're here," he said exhaustedly. "I'll be waiting for your calls. Any surprises and I'll be back here in four hours. Less if I can charter a plane."

"Do you think I can do everything I need to do here? Do you think I can watch over him like I should?"

"Of course," he said, pulling me to him and holding me close. "You know what to look for now. You've got your mother instincts turned on. And Danny and Grace will be here. I have to go now. One kiss . . ."

He got out and lingered for a moment, leaning in the open window on the passenger side. "It's been one hell of a week, hasn't it?"

I hated to see him go.

"It will be all right, dear. Keep me posted on every detail."

"Meticulous care, meticulous care," I repeated.

"You got it. Love you."

Through the glass walls I watched him blend into the stream of businessmen leaving home after the weekend. What was he doing? Leaving home? Going home? Neither? Both?

17

Suspended

The early sunlight through the southeastern windows brightened the unit. It was 6:30 A.M. and already Danny was sorting through stacks of charts. Looking rested after his time off, the white of his crisply starched coat contrasted cleanly with the blackness of his hair. Everything about him had the crisp atmosphere of a clear beginning, a renewal.

I prayed it was a sign, a good omen.

"We're so glad to be back up here and even happier you're on duty again. Marnix asked me to give this to you."

He took the thank you note I handed him and read it.

"Thanks," Danny said. He folded the note and tucked it into his pocket.

"Well." I didn't know where to begin. So much had happened in Danny's absence. "Damion's made it through two tough rounds while you were gone. The heart and then a perforation."

"Yes, a difficult week. Let me review things. I'll talk to John Kelton and call your husband, too. Then I'll come in to talk to you and Damion about where we go from here. Dr. Brodsky will be doing an echocardiogram to see how Damion's doing postoperatively. We can talk about that and this morning's chest x-ray and the rest of the day's plans once I get a few things done."

I looked around. Every cubicle was occupied. Little Marty's legs kicked playfully in the space behind me. The two-year-old was back from a successful intestinal repair. On the right I saw that the preemie hadn't budged from under its blanket of tubes and gauze. And the other side of the unit was busy, too.

"Whenever you get time, Danny. But can I ask you one quick question? Do you think Damion looks good?"

I knew not having seen Damion for six days would give him a clearer perspective than ours.

"He keeps hanging in there," Danny answered with an encouraging expression.

I would have to be satisfied with that.

Slowly I walked into Damion's cubicle. "Dad said to say good morning to you, D. He's already at the office trying to get some work done."

"How long did his flight take?" Damion asked.

"Really fast. Less than an hour to Tallahassee. Dad couldn't see it last night because it was dark, but he said the flight path is neat. It goes right along the coastline so you can see the Gulf and the land at the same time."

Damion loved flying. He loved Space Camp, airplanes, everything about aeronautics.

He was more alert these days. I could see that he listened, and although he didn't have the energy to ask many questions, he seemed to enjoy hearing people talk to him again.

We continued talking about the flights for a few minutes until I noticed Damion getting tired.

"Pup, you take a nap. We have a lot to look forward to when Aunt Grace gets here this afternoon. You've got some tests scheduled later this morning, too. I'll tilt the blinds for you."

It was incredible. Three nights before, my head on Marnix's lap, I had been certain Damion would die. In the waiting room I had accepted death's inevitability. And now here we were this morning with me chattering on about airlines.

Thank God for letting him live and talk and think! When my surprise wears off, maybe I can rebuild my faith that he will live, but never so immoderately or so foolishly as before.

The acceptance of Damion's impending death a few nights ago had changed everything. I knew it now: we were not entitled to conversations with our children. We were not entitled to their intellects, their health, or even their lives. We had no right to demand these things. They were only gifts, generous loans extended to oblivious people like me. There was no guarantee that this latest and most merciful rescue would last. I knew that now; I'd learned it thoroughly. It was a lesson I wouldn't forget.

WEDNESDAY AFTERNOON

It had been a morning of assessment and testing. In the afternoon the doctors deciphered the test results for me.

"Very satisfactory." It was the first note of enthusiasm I had yet heard in Dr. Brodsky's voice. "I don't see any functional problem, and there is no evidence of any constrictive pericarditis after his strip."

"Oh, that's great. So the enlarged heart silhouette has no clinical meaning? We can relax?"

"I think so," he said pensively. "He looks clear. Damion, we'll do another echo on you in a week or two just to check. But you look like you fought your way out of this problem like a champ."

The chest x-ray report that I called into Marnix gave less cause for celebration. "This is from a study done early this morning. 'There is early pulmonary vascular congestion. The left lower lobe infiltrate is unchanged from prior x-rays. Pulmonary vasculature is slightly more prominent than yesterday.' That's it. How much do we have to be concerned about this congestion and fluid overload?"

"I don't know," Marnix said. "I'll talk to Danny about it when he calls."

"There's more. Remember earlier I told you Danny was going to send him down for a Doppler of the lower extremities to rule out deep vein thrombosis? This will make you and John happy. I got the sonogram report and Danny says he will talk with you about it. It says there is no evidence of thrombosis. No clots, Marnix. Is that due to the heparin, do you suppose?"

"We'll never know, but it certainly didn't hurt. We can't relax on this. Keep trying to move his legs around for him. Do those bending exercises we've been working on."

"We are. And Danny ordered special stockings that compress his legs."

"Good. Keep them on him."

"And here is the last report, an abdominal x-ray. It revealed 'scattered collections of gases and some irregularity in the contours of the bowel loops with minor thumb printing.'" I put the papers down on the bed. "That's all I have for you so far. Dr. Kiros said he's doing well and he heard some bowel sounds. However, the diarrhea's still there, which is amazing when you think about it: he's had nearly a month of diarrhea. I don't know where it can keep coming from. His belly is still distended like yesterday, but everyone says that's due to gas and the manipulation of surgery. All in all, Kiros basically liked what he saw."

"That's really good. Every day that goes by without another perforation makes the outlook brighter."

"There's one last thing I want to mention to you," I said. "This term thumb printing. Remember Dr. Nicoletto picked it up at the other hospital on the gastrograph? Well, here it is again today. One of the articles in the packet we got from Mitchell talks about thumb printing being one of the distinctive markers of O-one-five-seven:H-seven infection."

"Interesting."

"More than that, it's consistent!" I felt the passion rising in my voice. "It's one more piece of the puzzle, a perfect fit like all the others to show us how this all happened to Damion. We have yet to come up with anything that isn't consistent with this strange pathogen, you notice that?"

Marnix listened without comment. He was still allowing me to pursue this research alone. I suspected this would continue until Damion was out of the woods. It was like crying over spilled milk from his point of view.

But for me, there was nothing plaintive about what I was doing each time I reread the medical literature late at night in the parent lounge. My search was born of nothing more than vengeance. I was angry about what had happened to our son. It was as though Damion had been run over and left bloodied on the road. I couldn't help him like Marnix and all the expert doctors but I could find out who was the evil culprit allowed to drive freely along our highways mowing down children at random.

Marnix was quiet perhaps because he suspected I was

embarking on a foolhardy mission. I knew I had no medical training. But I was Damion's mother and I was angry, and I was becoming more determined to find and root out the evil which had struck our son.

"Well, listen. I know you're swamped. I'll let you get back to seeing patients and will call you this evening with his numbers again. I wish you were here, Marnix."

"Me too. Call me around six if you can. And watch that temp."

"I'll do my best. You talk to Danny about the antibiotic coverage. As I said, he's very busy but he did say he'd call you soon."

MONDAY NIGHT

"So, Grace. You've got to be honest with me. What do you think? How does Damion look to you?"

She paused and then blinked in her honest way.

"Like he's been through a war. Which he has."

"Do you think he looks really bad? I mean, worse than you expected?"

She shook her head. "No. But he's very tired, just as I would expect. You have to understand he's had the life nearly kicked out of him."

"I know. How do you mean he looks very tired?"

I knew this was a ridiculous conversation but Grace was a nurse and my big sister, and I couldn't help wanting her to fix things. Her opinion was important.

"I mean, what did he do that made you think he's really tired?"

"Everything really. He has little pulmonary reserve. When he talks, he gets out of breath. And you know how he likes to talk. If he had his usual energy, he'd be firing questions at me about David, Jessica and Sarah."

"Yeah. He doesn't have much to say, but he *is* interested again. A week or two ago he wasn't," I defended.

We were in the parent room, and Grace produced a bottle of wine from her carry-on. It was about the last thing I'd ever think of, but it looked inviting. Grace sat Indian style on Marnix's bed while I sat on mine. We made a mess of a bath towel trying to punch down the cork with a plastic knife from the cafeteria. Finally we got the cork out and she poured some for each of us into plastic cups.

"The thing is," she went on, "he looks appropriately terrible for all he's been through. He's put up a tough fight and made it through some brutal things. It's going to take a long time to pull him together again. But you will."

"You don't think another major assault may be brewing? That this is just one more quiet period before a new storm?"

"I don't know." She shook her head and sipped some wine, then continued. "It looks to me more like he's getting into the knitting back together period. At least, let's hope so."

I sipped the wine, thinking how alike and yet dissimilar our lives were now.

"Is this a sin?" I asked.

"What? Drinking on a pediatric ward in a Catholic hospital?"

"Everyone knows that's a *venial* one! I'm talking about pouring good wine into plastic cups. Doesn't the Baltimore Catechism list that as a mortal sin?"

She laughed. "I won't tell Auntie Grace if you don't." Auntie Grace was our mom's sister who'd entered the Ursuline convent at sixteen years of age. She remained there her entire life. Grace was named after her.

"Don't make me feel guilty. You know how I've told you this place has been wonderful to us. This is a hospital with a mission."

"Toast. Here's to St. Joseph's for helping Damion." She raised her cup.

I lifted mine. "And here's to being exhausted."

Grace looked at me strangely.

"I'm too tired now to explain, but I will try over the next few days." I started undressing and putting on a nightgown. It seemed to me the stage of exhaustion would naturally follow the complications-will-kill-you phase. And it would have to precede the plateau of putting our lives back together again. Tonight I dared not propose a toast to more than one level of progress at a time.

Please let us be arriving at the point of exhaustion. Let us already be there.

"Prosit, Grace. Thanks for coming."

I crawled under the covers and fell into immediate sleep.

TUESDAY, MARCH 24

Mid morning light sliced into our room through the tilted slats of the blinds. "Oh, for crying out loud," I cried when I saw the clock read after nine. I leapt from bed, amazed and ashamed. Where was Grace? Throwing on an overly worn yellow blouse and the same navy pants that were permanently stretched and molded to my form, I washed my face, brushed my teeth and hair and rushed out of the room.

How could I have slept more than eight hours, I wondered as I hurried. It wasn't the wine: I'd only had two cups. Grace's bed was not even rumpled. Where was she?

I found her in the unit standing with Terri beside Damion's bed.

"Sorry, D., to be so late. Grace, never let me oversleep like that again. What's going on here? Hi, Terri. You've obviously met my sister Grace."

"We've been at it for hours. We've done all kinds of things. Right, guys?"

"Gosh, sorry you all. I must have been really zonked. And what happened to your NG tube, D.?" I asked, suddenly noticing its absence. The only tube under his nose was the small band of plastic attached to the oxygen tank.

"It's gone," he answered happily. "Danny pulled it out this morning. He said I could try to drink fluids again, and that it was time to get my stomach working."

"Damion, that's great!"

"I already had an Italian ice, a lemon one. In an hour I get to try a strawberry one."

"Terrific!" I patted his hand and tried not to think of his drinking the strawberry Slurpy four days before.

He seemed happy, almost anticipatory. His glasses were on, and he wore his favorite blue Umbros that I kept rinsing out for him. The surgical dressing was still taped over his belly. The chest incision above the dressing was knitting back together into a shiny red line. Every day its dressing was made smaller, revealing more and more of its length.

Grace smiled at me and said, "Last night you were tossing so much that I thought I was bothering you. So I snuck out and slept in the parent lounge. I came in and out to sit with D. through the night."

"Then you need your sleep now."

"No, I'm in good shape. Well, Terri, is it time?"

Terri, more upbeat than even her usual positive self, said, "Let's do it! Are you ready, Damion?"

"We were waiting for you," he told me as if they were about to spring a wonderful surprise.

"What are you all up to?"

"This," Terri said as she and Grace pulled Damion upright into a crouched sitting position on his bed. His spine was bent from being curled in an almost fetal position for a month. When he had lain on his back, the back of his bed was kept elevated to help his lungs drain. He had never been flat, and now he looked frozen into his new shape as surely as my pants conformed to me.

Terri and Grace swiveled Damion's bony legs around so that they dangled off the side of the bed.

"Sit there a minute until you don't feel lightheaded. Let you body adjust and then we'll do it."

"Can I have my shoes on?"

"Wow!" I exclaimed as I rushed out to retrieve his black Nikes and socks from their storage place under my bed. While I put his socks and shoes on, Grace pushed the IV poles away and gathered up his lines and tubes. She got on Damion's left and Terri got on his right. They pulled him to a standing position.

"Wow, D.!" I laughed. "You are standing! You really are standing!"

"Okay, three steps. We won't let go. Go real slow. Now let us turn you a little bit."

They swiveled Damion 45 degrees and then gently lowered him into the recliner they had prepared. He sat as erectly as he could and as proudly as if he had just won the state soccer tournament.

"I'm so proud of you! You look absolutely fantastic!"

Happiness flowed through me. There was something about him being out of bed that made him appear less sick and vulnerable. He was advancing, no doubt about it. Danny heard all the commotion and came in to look.

"Very good, Damion," he exclaimed. "How does it feel? At first it's a little strange, but this is good for you. I want you to try to sit there twenty or thirty minutes today. We'll build up the time each day. It will help your lungs, make you stronger, and prevent you from forming clots. He looks terrific, doesn't he, Mom?"

"Powerful!" I answered, tears rising in my eyes.

"So let's get the camera," Grace suggested. She grabbed the Polaroid from the window ledge, got us posed, and shot some pictures. "You know, I bet the hospital will fax this to your dad if we ask," she said as an image emerged.

"Sure, we can do that," Terri agreed. "First, we'll blow it up on the copier so it will transmit better and he can see the detail. He wouldn't want to miss this."

"Good idea," I said. "He will love this when it comes off his fax machine."

AFTERNOON

Damion was able to sit in the chair twenty minutes before he became so tired that he asked to get back to bed. Almost immediately, he fell into a long nap, but getting out of bed represented great progress. His chest x-ray was also encouraging compared to yesterday's. I reported our progress to Marnix and was hardly able to contain the hope springing back to life within me.

The news was not universally good. "The left lower lobe remains a problem. It's been a problem since the cardiopulmonary mess began. But at least the right lung is looking better today," I told Marnix.

"And they always do the percussion on him after the breathing treatments?"

"Always. They pound on his left back at least ten minutes."

"Good. We've got to get that consolidation loosened up. And make sure he does his best blowing into the inspirometer. He's got to get all these little segments filled back up with air."

"He uses it every time they come up for a treatment. They are very demanding of him in a pleasant way."

"Good. You should make him do it every couple of hours, too."

I told Marnix about the persistent fever and Dr. Kiros's visit and his report to me that Damion might be developing an intestinal shutdown. Damion's gastrointestinal tract had been so insulted by the infection, weeks of lying dormant, and the perforation and trauma of surgery that it was now shutting down.

"Intestines do not like to be handled," Marnix said. "They go on strike."

"Dr. Kiros said it may be days before Damion can go from fluids to eating food. We just have to wait until his system gets over everything and wakes back up. Even Damion's intestines are in a state of exhaustion, I think."

"I'm glad Danny's being aggressive with that fever," Marnix said, changing the topic. "I knew this loomed as a larger concern than the timing of his G.I. tract being turned on."

"Yes. They are constantly shooting antibiotics into Damion's IV's. By the way, did you get your surprise?"

"Surprise?" he repeated suspiciously. "What are you talking about?"

"Call upstairs to Phyllis and see if something's on the fax for you. I'll be here a few minutes if you want to call back and talk about it."

To Marnix at this point, no news was good news and the only surprises we'd been having were bad ones. "Don't worry, Marnix. It's something from Damion to you."

After I'd hung up, I noticed Grace had done some washing of my laundry that had been piling up. As I was smoothing out the clean laundry on my bed, the phone rang.

"Mary, I'm shocked." Marnix's voice was low.

"Yeah, can you believe it? It's great."

"Great? It's shocking," he said in a depressed tone.

"How can you be discouraged by him sitting upright?"

"That's not it. I'm glad to see him up, but I couldn't see it when I left. Do you see how emaciated he is? All that's left is bone."

I stretched the phone cord over to the dresser and looked down at the photo of Damion. Marnix was right. It was unbelievable how wasted Damion looked. In all the excitement of Damion's effort and pride in sitting up, I hadn't really looked at him, I realized.

"Do me a favor," Marnix asked. "Talk to Danny, and I will, too. We've got to see if we can crank up his TPN and add more protein, especially if it'll be days yet before he can eat."

"I will, Marnix."

"I never saw it until now," he said fearfully. "He is starving."

WEDNESDAY, MARCH 25

Damion was feverish and complaining of pain in his belly and was too tired to sit in the chair. Despite all our encouragement to sit, it seemed too much for him.

"My muscles are aching. Can I just do this twice as long tomorrow instead?"

Danny sat on the edge of Damion's bed.

"Okay, Damion. Radiology will be up to take more pictures of your belly. I want to know why I hear no bowel sounds with my stethoscope. We'll see how you feel this afternoon. Maybe then you'll feel like sitting up a few minutes."

"Thanks. I'll try then," Damion promised and scrunched down in the bed.

Walking out to the desk with him, I asked Danny if he thought Damion simply did too much yesterday.

"He's sore and worn out," Danny explained, "not only from the effort, but perhaps from the continuing fever. It could be attributable to something I've been suspecting: an abdominal obstruction." He said he hoped another x-ray series would reveal the problem. Was it only an ileus? Or could it be a blockage? Why was Damion's abdomen so rigid? Why did he have so much pain when pressure was applied to his lower quadrants? Why was he still running a fever?

X-rays were soon shot of his abdomen and chest. An hour later, the reports were ready. I called the news into Marnix. "No significant change."

"Okay," Marnix said. "Sounds like everything has come to a halt, but I think we might be okay here. No free air to show a perforation, no visible obstruction. The question is that fever. With the massive umbrella of antibiotics he's under, the fever is just so darn perplexing."

"Maybe post-op? Don't people often run a fever because of operative trauma? It seems hard to believe he's cooking up a big infection somewhere. I know he had the fecal spillage from the perforation but isn't he under the big guns as far as antibiotics go?"

"Yes, he is. This is confusing. I know that Danny's worried about it, and the infectious disease fellow can't come up with anything."

No surprise there, I thought.

"Did you talk to Danny about the TPN and the possibility of adding more calories and protein?"

The photo that frightened Marnix was still at the top of my papers. *Skeletal, he does look skeletal. You are absolutely right, Marnix. This is a scary picture.*

"Basically I think he feels there's only so much we can do until he can start eating again. Danny is doing all he can."

"I know he is. I'm just feeling like you do that there are only so many days we have. Obviously, his expenditures are exceeding his intake. He can't go on like this forever."

Then Marnix asked, "What about his chest? You have that report?"

"Yes. Oh, and this one sounds very good to me. I hope you agree: 'Aeration of the lungs has improved, and there is significantly less atelectasis. Upper lungs are clear.' Nice, huh? The word 'improved' sounds good. Is it respiratory therapy that's making the difference?"

"I don't know. But this is good news. It makes me feel that the congestion of two days ago might be resolving. That might even have been a mistaken impression by the radiologist."

"Oh good, good, good. Do you want to speak to Grace? She's with Damion. She can go over all the blood work with you. It's all unchanged since yesterday."

Marnix indicated he did. "Hold on," I said and went to get Grace.

MID AFTERNOON

On my way to the mail room to pick up a package sent by John Kelton, I thought of how a hospital was like a town in microcosm. In it was an automatic teller machine, the gift shop, the information desk, cafeteria, and many other services including a chapel. I'd yet to go to the chapel. I'd developed almost a superstition about it. Somehow it seemed melodramatic that a mother would come down here to plead for her child's life. I felt I'd found a better place for prayer on the eighth floor where I felt closer to the grand designer of the universe.

Past the cafeteria I took a staircase to the basement. I knew my way through the network of corridors linking laundry, shipping, supplies, receiving, and the mail room. I always chose the long way around to the post office, because of the morgue.

Each of us carries around a pocket full of images from our childhood, some of which are happy while others are disturbing. My most vividly shocking image came from a mistake I once made. On a class trip to the National Institutes of Health, I took the wrong hallway back to my tenth grade group. Passing through untraveled corridors, I peered through a window cut into a metal door and saw an autopsy of a young child in progress. I'll never forget the glimpse of an opened belly, bloated limbs, and the surprisingly yellow color of fat highlighted against the green tiled walls. It remained an ugly snapshot etched in my memory.

One day I nearly made a similar mistake here. Walking casually on the most direct path to the mail room, I found myself passing in front of swinging doors marked Morgue. Scenes flashed through my mind of my childhood encounter. Ever since, I avoided that hallway very carefully.

The nice woman in the mail room sold me stamps, gave me boxes if I needed them, and always asked about Damion. "He must be a popular guy for all the mail he gets each day," she smiled. "Be sure to bring him down when he feels better so we can meet him."

On the way back upstairs holding John Kelton's package, I reflected on the condensed world now enfolding us in the hospital. It was almost as if I'd never lived in the real one.

NIGHT

"Grace, I hate your going home tomorrow without any resolution about Damion. It's frustrating to me that not only are we stuck in this state of limbo here, but now you're leaving and nothing is resolved. His G.I. problem remains. The fever is a continuing mystery. Other than him sitting up yesterday, I see no progress you can take home with you."

"I can," Grace said. "He's more tuned in than when I came. I don't agree with you that there's no discernible progress."

"I just want to know when and how he's going to pull out of this period. We're just stuck here."

"But remember where he was a week ago. That was a very scary time with Damion coming out of heart surgery. This is dramatic progress."

I sighed. "You're right. At the very least, the last few days have been a respite. I should accept them on that basis. We'll know the future soon enough."

"It's going to take a long time, but I think it's going to work out," my big sister said seriously.

As I stuffed the pillow under my head, I thought about how much help and comfort Grace had been. I'd miss her watching over the numbers, I'd miss the time she spent with Damion, our talks, and most of all her unwavering assurance that it would work out.

"I'm really glad you came. It's like your visit came at a time when we are suspended in the air above an ocean of damage. I admit this makes little sense, and I'm not saying it well, but that's what the days of your visit have felt like. Like we're stranded here on a dizzying ride through space but momentarily safe. Anyway, you helped a lot by coming now."

"That was the idea. You get a good night's sleep. I'll go read by him for a couple of hours."

"Oh, Grace, thanks."

I turned over and, before I fell asleep, I wondered how we would get from this suspended place in space back to the real safety of solid ground.

18

Unforeseen Turn

"Mom, look. Watch it with me. That lady and man are Bobby Hurley's parents. You know the Duke player that was in the game Dad and I watched, the short one? That was Bobby Hurley. The father's a high school coach and they have another son named Danny who's a player for Seton Hall. Both brothers always played on the same high school team together but they have to play against each other tonight."

"You're kidding. Wouldn't that be difficult? Could you ever play against Sebastian in a big game?"

"Mm hum," he nodded, not taking his eyes off the television program.

"Well, I'd hate to be their mom. The only thing I could hope for would be a tie. They do have ties in college basketball, don't they?"

Damion was very patient with my lack of sports knowledge. Politely, he didn't respond. I could do better, I know, but there was no incentive. Marnix had orchestrated that part of the boys' lives: coaching their teams, playing rousing soccer matches in the back-yard with them before dinner, creating excitement by hauling out special snacks and cranking the volume up to stadium level when-ever a major event was televised. It was their thing. I thought that by having a daughter she and I could do our thing during the boys' sports activities, but that plan had been foiled by her dad fashion-ing her into a jock as well. So whenever it was NCAA champi-onships, World Series, or Stanley Cup season, I wandered off and enjoyed the gift of quiet time.

When the interview with Mr. and Mrs. Hurley ended, I lifted the magical Duke cap off the pole where a nurse had clipped it and pulled out the diagram folded inside.

Damion's expression told me that he took this seriously.

"Have you seen Dr. Plasencia yet? He must still be on the other side of the unit. What's up so far today? Has the x-ray machine been in?"

"Yep. Danny said I'm going to go downstairs for a CAT scan later this morning."

"Oh really? Did he say why?"

"He's still wondering about why I can't eat yet and wants to see if I have an obstruction. The only bad thing about the test is that I have to drink this disgusting fluid with barium in it. I have to start drinking four cups of that gook at 10:00. It's to light up my intestines so they will glow in the dark."

I grimaced. "It might not taste so great but they'll probably mix it with juice to make it better. The main thing is that it will be good to get a clear picture of your insides to make sure they are healing the right way. And Grace and I will come with you today. It will be cool to see how the technology works."

"Do I get to see the pictures it makes?"

"I don't see why not; it's your belly. I'm sure Danny will show you everything."

Within a couple of hours Damion had consumed four ten-ounce Styrofoam cups of orange flavored liquid. It was an effort to drink that much, but he managed to keep it down. Grace and I were allowed to push him and his IV poles down to Radiology. She asked Danny if we could wheel Damion outside onto a patio for a few minutes after the scan.

"Sure, get some fresh air."

After the hour or so that it took in Radiology we found an empty courtyard.

"Our first time outside! What a beautiful cool spring day for you, D."

We parked the wheelchair under a willow that fragmented the strong sunlight into a thousand serrated shadows across his thin face. He blinked sleepily and didn't focus on anything specific within the small courtyard. His face wore the same expression it did

when he was a blanketed baby on our strolls. He had the same diffuse awareness of swaying branches, the same dreamy submersion
in patterns of sun and leaves that inevitably caused his heavy head
to fall against the carriage rails. Soon this happened here. Grace slid
a pillow between his fallen head and the wheelchair frame. He dozed
peacefully under the baby blue hospital blanket. She read one of
her books. I sat on the patch of grass, against the willow's trunk,
and dreamed of that simple time. Those blissful infant days had
scrolled by slowly for Marnix and me, as slowly as our stroller
wheels against the asphalt eleven years ago. Baby sleeping. Sunlight,
shade and gladness drifting up and down our oak lined street.

"What do you say we get him back upstairs?" I asked Grace
after thirty minutes. "He's exhausted."

AFTERNOON

The report from the CAT scan must have beaten us back
upstairs. As Grace and his nurse settled Damion back into bed,
Danny took me aside to tell me the findings.

"We still can't tell what is going on in Damion's belly. We'll
have to take him back to the O.R.

My face fell. "Oh, not again. Not another crisis. Oh man, how
many does this make?" Counting the catheter implant, the pericardial strip, the perforation, and the taps, this would be the seventh
procedure Damion had to endure. Seven. Was the number seven
portentous? Good luck or bad? How were we going to tell him?

To my surprise, when we did, Damion was more worried
about his television schedule than what was about to happen again.
"Will I be back upstairs in time to watch the game?"

Despite my fears I had to smile. The flexibility of children
and their ability to adapt was amazing in such circumstances as
these. How blessed he was. While we adults steeled ourselves thinking we cannot endure it, children accept the inevitable and move on.

"Yes," Danny assured him. "Dr. Swank will take you in
another hour, Damion. I'm going to come in the operating room
and stay with you. It won't take a long time."

"And no respirator when I wake up?"

"I think by the time you come out of Recovery, it will be out.
This is going to be a lot easier than the last one. It will be a small

incision, maybe only big enough for a scope to enter. We're looking for something like a pool of fluid in your belly. We know what to do if we find it. The anesthesia won't be so heavy. Yes, we'll get you back up here for the game."

"Good."

Danny turned to me. "Do you have any questions?"

"Only, Danny, would you mind calling Marnix about it?"

"Yes, of course. I'll call him now. Any other questions? Damion? Well then, I'll call your papa."

"You heard from Danny, didn't you?" It was a rhetorical question. Marnix's tone of voice told me he already knew.

"Did Danny read to you the CAT scan report?"

"No. He discussed it though. Do you have it with you?"

"Yes. I'll fax it to you. So Danny went over with you about how this is most likely an abscess and how he'll stay in surgery with Damion to see himself what's going on inside him?"

"Let's hope it's as simple as an abscess. That would be the best choice out of things like obstruction and perforation. The thing that bothers me is that the majority of abscesses are infected. You just never know until you go in."

"Did Danny tell you Damion's one concern going into this surgery?"

"Yeah, sweet boy. I hope he can get back up in time for the game."

"Marnix, are we just getting inured to this? Here Damion's on his way back to the operating room: and you and I are not choking with fear. Damion's only wondering if it will mess up Duke's chances of advancing to the Final Four. It seems like an abnormal reaction. Maybe we've just been here too long." I gave a heavy sigh.

He said nothing.

EVENING

Danny called for me sooner than I expected. His expression was relieved when he described the pocket of fluid they found and aspirated in the lower section of Damion's abdomen.

"It was a puddle. The same fluid we've found in him before: clear, serous, odorless fluid, much like what we kept tapping from his pericardial sac. There was no pus, thank goodness, although we'll have to wait for the lab to say conclusively if it was sterile."

"Was it a lot? Enough to account for all the bloating?"

"Yes, a very substantial collection on both sides of his colon extending down into the pelvis and filling up most of the deeper part of his pelvic space. After it was aspirated, Dr. Swank sewed a drain in place."

"Danny, do you think this abscess is secondary to the perforation?"

"We don't know. It very well could be connected. I hope removing it puts an end to Damion's temperature and ileus."

"When do you think I can see him?"

"Now. He's already been extubated. He's still coming out from under the anesthesia, but he'll ask for you in a few minutes. I thought I'd come and get you before he has to ask."

"I'm really glad you stayed with him. I bet he was, also," I said as we pushed against the Recovery Room doors.

"It helped me, too. I had to see what was going on."

We entered the room.

"Damion, your mom is here. Can you hear me? You did very well, Damion. Dr. Swank has you all set, and we're going to try and get you back upstairs in time like we promised, okay? As soon as we can, we'll take you up."

NIGHT

By the time Damion was settled back in the unit, the Duke game was just getting underway. Within moments he was reattached to the monitor and all his lines. Then the nurses let him watch television. For the next hour and a half, Damion tried to stay awake. He explained to me the good defense played by both Duke and Seton Hall, and concentrated on touching certain parts of his cap during particular plays. The game was close. Duke led 48-44.

"Damion, isn't this a little nerve wracking? There's only fifteen more minutes to go and it's been neck and neck the whole time. They might tie after all!"

"Don't worry," he said confidently, still not telling me there is no such thing as a tie in college basketball.

He focused on every move, never taking his attention away

from the screen. He kept touching his Duke hat. He's out there with them, I thought. He's totally immersed in their strategy and fight.

"What's going on when you rub the brim like that?"

"That's for rebounding. See, they're pulling ahead now. They must have been saving it for the end."

Duke ended up winning 81-69. Damion listened to Bobby Hurley in a post-game interview when he said, "When my brother was out there it was a weird situation. It was real distracting. It was the hardest thing I had to do all year."

Damion was now very tired and had begun to doze off.

"Well, D.D., you and Bobby Hurley did it. You got through another big round of your own today. Good work, big boy. I'll hang this back up on the suction thing where you can see it. This is quite a lucky hat Dr. Kelton sent."

"Night, Mom," he said sleepily.

"Good night, darling. I'm so proud of you. And Duke, too," I remembered to add.

After he fell asleep, I wandered out into the hall past the premature baby on the respirator, past Marty and an empty space. This was the extent of my exercise program here: walking past all the sleeping pediatrics rooms, circling the elevator core, and ending up at the parent lounge where no one would see me stretch and bend. Then I would look out on the cityscape and pray.

A lighted pyramid atop one of the tallest buildings of the skyline seemed a beacon. Its lights were timed to turn off at 3:00 A.M., but until then it glowed across the night. The concrete building was as strong and constant as a lighthouse at sea. I'd come to love this building and its calming influence. All my scattered prayers were collected and focused into a more coherent pleading when I fixated on its triangular whiteness.

Sometimes I wondered if I'd ever see it from the daytime streets below. Would I ever stand at the base of its shadow and think about the outcome of all this?

Many nights I was too tired to do any more than watch the structure and remember. The white translucence of the triangular pediment reminded me of nine months before when the moonlight bathed a happy night. Damion and his friends had been jumping off our ancient dock into the warm June lake. Frogs were calling and the boys were bobbing sleek as beavers in the darkening water. Robust bodies hoisted themselves up the wooden ladder to mount the diving board again. There they stood, water puddling at their feet, anxious for the boy jumping ahead of them to paddle out of the way. Damion's torso arched and glowed in the moonlight.

Now, once again I saw his luminous body, milky as it slid into the dark velvet water. Then it was replaced by a white building, radiant against the wet black sky. A building and a boy. A building and a boy. My simple good night prayer was: *keep them bright.*

19

Lost Safety Net

Lucky seven. Could it be? Were we near the end, or would there be another complication, another dizzying precipitous turn or drop on this fearful ride?

The weekend was here. Marnix would be back at the hospital soon. We'd all pull up chairs to Damion's bed to watch and wait. Did the abscess account for Damion' temperature? Were the antibiotics covering all the microbial dangers? Would his intestines wake up? Would his left lower lung clear?

These were not the catastrophic complications we faced earlier; they were chronic, ongoing ones, but they could wear him down as surely as the dramatic hits, only insidiously, more slowly.

The doctors tried to categorize these stubborn problems one by one and search out their solutions, a still arduous and dangerous process. Then they had to repair the damage so Damion could begin to mend.

AFTERNOON

"Marnix, it's better with you here." He held me close.

"You don't know how hard it was to be away," he told me. "It's almost impossible to get through the week, imagining what's going on here. It's a big relief to see Damion. I think he looks pretty good." He stepped back.

"You mean it?" I asked, almost afraid to believe his words and look into his eyes.

We'd just come back to our little room together, after Marnix said hello to Damion and delivered a bundle of notes from the children at home.

"I do. He's thinner than when I left, but he's hanging in there. I'll tell you, the major blessing of the week is that he did not throw another clot somewhere. God, I'm so grateful for that."

"Right. No perforations, no stroke, no major disaster all week. Only the abscess."

"And they took care of that."

I thought aloud, taking inventory of Damion's status, "Seems like his lungs are a problem that won't let up. Can you ask Danny about this morning's x-ray? It mentioned pneumonia."

Marnix bent down and picked up his overnight bag and walked over to the bureau zipping it open. He pulled out his radio and shaver and stacked up note pads on the bureau. He tossed a box on my bed. "Here's the stationery you asked for. I've already talked to Danny. He doesn't think it's bacterial or viral pneumonia. I think he's right."

"Why do you think his lung is so slow to mend? I could see it when he had fluid backing up all the time, but now why are his lungs continuing to weep fluid?"

"This appears to be old damage. If you think about the disease process, a logical explanation would be his lung could have been hit by a clot or a shower of mini clots that knocked out that section of tissue."

"You think so? Has Danny or John talked with you about this clot theory?"

"No. Danny is perplexed by the persistence of the problem. John and I haven't talked specifically about an embolus to the lung. But the more I think of it, the more sense it makes."

Marnix was anxious to get back to the unit. But first he handed me a list of who had done what for us back in Dothan.

SATURDAY MORNING, MARCH 28

Damion felt sick to his stomach and uncomfortable. So Danny decided to put the NG tube back in. Damion wasn't able to eat anyway, and remembering how it had helped his nausea before, he did not object.

"Until this ileus and the gas on x-ray clears up, you'll feel better with this tube again, Damion," Danny explained. Again the tea colored fluid was drawn from Damion's stomach, up into the vacuum canister on the wall.

For now the TPN would have to continue to keep him fed. I remained grateful to this wire threaded under his shoulder and through a vein feeding into his heart's right atrium. The nutrition dripped like it had all month now.

This morning the suspended bottle of lipids also dripped onto our floor and under his bed. "What's this stickiness up close to his bed?" I traced the spill back and found the dripping line.

The nurse reclamped the connections. "I'll call housekeeping. This is too big a mess to wipe up with paper towels."

Soon Maria came in to mop up. She looked furtively at Damion sleeping and his father reading as she wrung out her floor mop in a pail of disinfectant. Then she winked to me as though we had a secret pact. I smiled back. She was very shy compared to the times she cornered me alone. Marnix swung his long legs aside when he saw he was in the way.

"Sorry. Oh, here, let me move the bed for you." He jumped up to help her.

She cleaned under the bed very determinedly.

"Thank you for mopping that up for us," he said.

This emboldened Maria to say, "He look very nice this morning. He getting better now."

"Thank you. We hope so." Marnix wasn't aware of how deeply she watched and cared.

"Definitely he getting better. I look at heem every day. Dees I'm chore of."

SUNDAY, LATE AFTERNOON

Before Marnix went home on that Sunday evening, we left Damion alone to go for a long walk together. Terri and another nurse had brought their own eleven and twelve-year-old boys over to watch *Top Gun* with Damion in the P.I.C.U. Upon introduction, these two young visitors seemed surprised and maybe a bit frightened by Damion's appearance. But soon they overlooked it and began watching the movie with him. We left them sitting awkwardly and doing what unacquainted boys this age do, talking little with one other, but generally pleased to be in each other's company.

"It's so nice of the nurses to bring their boys. He misses being with kids his age. This is really good for him today," I said, taking the arm Marnix extended.

"Let's talk about the week ahead," Marnix suggested. "There are still some important things that must be done if we're to get Damion on the way to recovery. Obviously, we've got to get this ileus resolved. He needs to get going with his own intake."

"When he does, can he stay on TPN at the same time? Overlap a little until he can take in enough calories and protein on his own?"

"Once he can eat, Danny will probably take the central venous line out as soon as possible. Remember part of John's advice with respect to meticulous care: 'Lines out! As soon as you can, lines out! Guard against infection.' You're going to have to continue staying right on top of his dressing changes and IV's."

"But the nurses are doing that conscientiously."

"I know, they're great, but if someone new comes in, or if someone gets too busy one day, you don't know how many things can happen in a hospital. You just need to maintain the same kind of vigilance you and Grace did last week. Watch his numbers, watch the dressings. Don't forget where we are in the disease. This is when you can still lose him on a technicality."

"I know, I know. Do you think we're getting anywhere clearing his lungs?"

"That's another big one for the week ahead. I'm glad Danny will be on all week. He's very focused on this concern. Respiratory Therapy is really getting aggressive with Damion now. We have to keep that up. I know the treatments tire him out, but that's all he's got to do now. Try to encourage him to sit up and use the inspirometer. He's got to force air into all those little segments that have collapsed. He's trying very hard but he's got a long way to go."

As we passed a sleek glass building for cardiac care, we looked up to the third story at a row of middle-aged men exerting themselves on Life Cycles. They were trying very hard, too.

"Well, I hate it that you have to leave again but I know it's good for the other kids when you're home. Do you know what makes me feel so guilty?"

"What?"

"I know this sounds horrible, but in retrospect I am glad that we are this far away from home. If Damion was hospitalized nearby, we couldn't have done it. There'd be a tug of war with thinking about all the other children's needs, not to mention visitors during the more grueling times when we couldn't have handled them. I think we needed to be this far away so we could concentrate entirely on him. Does that make any sense?"

"I know exactly what you mean. I agree we needed to put all our energy into helping Damion. This would have been impossible at home."

We were almost back to the front entrance. We wouldn't be able to talk like this again for days.

"So, Marnix, do you think the worst is over? Do you think he will make it now?"

"I think that much more so than two or three weeks ago. There's no guarantee, but if he can just stay away from infection and get over these last two complications, he will."

"And you think the damage will not be life impairing?"

"It's going to be a while before we can assess what his kidneys and lungs and neurological function lost, but remember what we prayed for. We asked only that we could take him home, which was asking a lot. If we're able to do that, we can figure out the rest later."

"You're right," I said.

"I'd better start getting ready to go soon. Can you check on my flight? That'll give me a few more minutes with him."

MONDAY MORNING, MARCH 30

Damion was undergoing a breathing treatment with Robert. First, a hose blew medicated mist into Damion's mouth. Then Robert used a cup-like object to pound gently on Damion's lower left side, the most stubborn quadrant to clear up. The idea of this percussion was to loosen any congestion and fluid so he could cough it up.

The pounding took ten minutes during which Robert teased Damion about Duke and Bobby Hurley. Damion could not respond with the little breath he had knocked out of him. Robert teased on, like a dentist talking while a patient was under the drill. At the end, Damion said only a confident, "Duke is going to win."

"There you go again! You've got to stop saying foolish things! Damion, if they can fend off Indiana in the Metrodome, I will crawl into your room and kiss your feet the next day before I begin your treatment. That's right, I will," he promised.

"Deal?" Damion extended his hand.

"Deal." Robert held it tenderly.

AFTERNOON

The days were settling into a routine. Sessions with Robert for respiratory therapy, Dr. Kiros's checks on the abdominal x-rays, and physical examinations. Smaller things like Damion's appearance that wouldn't have bothered us earlier now gained a certain amount of attention.

"Do you want me to try and get your hair cut, D.? Let me grab a mirror and let you see."

He looked at how long and limp his hair was.

"Or you could risk it and allow me to cut it."

"No way." I had one by one made a mess of my children's hair at some point so that none of them would allow me to approach them with scissors. The only exception was Mila and that was for bangs only.

"Let me see if someone can come up and do that for you."

The nurses contacted the barber who came to the hospital to cut patients' hair and the man came later that same afternoon.

This is good, I thought as I watched wisps of hair fall on his toweled shoulders. We must be getting somewhere if we're having his hair cut. I handed him the mirror when the cut was finished.

"You look good, D. Here, check yourself out and tell this gentleman if you want it shorter."

Seven is a lucky number. Isn't it? The words rolled around in my mind.

NIGHT

M.T. only seemed to appear at night. What does this funny young woman do in the daytime, I wondered.

"Saracita! Come see this!" she hollered toward our space. "I taught him a new trick!"

Sara's bemused response was to shake her head and smile.

"That M.T. is just a wild woman." She motioned me to follow her and said to Damion, "We'll tell you what she's up to in a minute."

Three or four other nurses and Dr. Sastry, who was on tonight, were already gathered around Marty's crib. M.T. pulled Marty up by his stocky arms and let his dimpled hands latch onto the rail of his crib. Then she stood back and commanded, "Okay, Marty. Not until I say the word."

Marty was wide-eyed in anticipation. He began to bounce on his legs but restrained himself, waiting for the countdown he knew would begin.

"Okay, Marty! Show them how! One. Two. Three. BOINK!"

On "BOINK!" Marty let go and fell back rigid as a tree trunk hard against his mattress. Proudly sprawled out, he waited for applause. Everyone clapped and laughed. I laughed at Marty's delighted expression as he waited for M.T. to pull him back up again and repeat the countdown.

"BOINK!" Over again he keeled, the respirator hose bouncing on his bare chest.

"Very good, very good," Dr. Sastry laughed approvingly.

The other nurses kissed Marty one by one as they filed back to resume their work. I gave him a hug, too, for showing me I had underestimated a child's resources and overestimated the burden of the respirator.

Sara went ahead of me to tell Damion about Marty's trick. When I came back into our space, he was laughing at the antics of a baby he'd never seen but who had become an intimate part of his life. In the days ahead, we'd hear an occasional slapping sound and smile at one another. It was Marty, who had managed to crawl up into position and was practicing his trick on his own.

"Way to go, Marty!" Damion would tell him.

TUESDAY, MARCH 31

The reports from Radiology kept showing the same gas patterns and the same atelectasis on every picture. Seeing no changes, Danny decided to forgo the daily x-rays for a couple of days. "We'll wait until tomorrow to do him again. Since we're seeing no clinical difference, let's limit some of the exposure he's getting."

This sounded good. In the back of my mind I was always

worried about the amount of radiation Damion was being bombarded with, necessary as it was.

"Danny, may I ask you about something Damion suggested? He wants to see if he can make it to his bathroom and take a tub bath."

Danny thought about this for a moment. I supposed he was considering all the lines and dressings and how many days it had been since the last abdominal incision was made. "I know it's ambitious, but Terri said she was going to change his dressings this morning. I wouldn't want him to do it if you think there's any risk, but that's what he asked for. I told him I'd ask you."

"If he keeps his hands and upper chest out of the water so the IV and subclavian lines aren't submerged that will be fine. And Terri with him the whole time."

"Okay. Thank you."

Damion balanced between both of us for the fifteen or so tedious steps it took to shuffle into the bathroom he'd never seen. He was so light that we essentially lifted him while he slowly put one foot in front of the other. Once inside, he asked if he could first use the toilet.

"Sure," Terri answered. "Your mom can help you on it, and then wait out here with me until you're done. Don't try to get up without us, okay? We'll give you a hand into the tub when you're ready."

The tub, thank goodness, amounted to a lip of tile no higher than twelve inches for him to step over.

"Okay," Damion answered as Terri stepped out.

To make undressing easier, Damion wore a hospital gown rather than his usual shorts or pair of scrubs. The gown had snaps at the shoulders to allow his lines to be threaded in the armholes. Only its top tie was fastened in back.

"Hold it a second, D. Let me get the pole out of the way for the door to shut. Hold on to me with your left hand, and the wall with your right."

In all the maneuvering I ended up behind him. His gown parted for a second or two. That's when I first saw what only standing could expose. It was astounding. Damion's backbone rose out from his flesh like a mountain chain. Each projection of every vertebra was defined. This bony range curved down till it terminated just above what used to be his buttocks and was now just the stark outline of his pelvic bones. I wanted to cry as he settled painfully onto the toilet seat.

I had no idea he'd reached this degree of emaciation. It was impossible to appreciate when he was laying down. Until he stood, I hadn't seen how ghastly his weight loss was.

"I'll wait in your room with Terri. Just tap on the door when you want us. See you in a few minutes."

I left him alone, glad he could reestablish the privacy so important to adolescents. The privacy he'd had to relinquish for so long.

20

Close to the Ground

WEDNESDAY MORNING, APRIL 1

It was time to read Marnix the reports from two x-rays taken this morning, both succinct and encouraging. We weren't there yet, but progress was clearly evident in today's films. There was slight improvement in the left lung, though some cloudiness still remained. And the views of the abdomen revealed some improvement with gas scattered throughout the colon. There were still some loops of small bowel with edema, though their appearance had improved over the last few days.

"Pretty good, huh?" I said to Marnix.

"Encouraging."

"And Danny says the fever curve has subsided."

"We've talked about that. It seems like last Thursday's drainage of the abscess finally cleaned it up."

I had caught Marnix between surgeries. I could visualize him standing by the large scrub sink between the two operating rooms. He would be propped against the wall with one paper-covered shoe kicking the other. The surgical nurses and the anesthesiologist would not press him to hurry. They knew he rarely took calls between cases, and it had to be important, so they'd wait patiently for him to finish.

"And Kiros and Danny feel he's ready to start on a simple diet. The NG tube is out, and they've ordered some kind of gruel and a Pediasure milk shake from downstairs. Damion's excited."

"Try to keep the TPN going for a couple more days. I think you'll find it's very hard for him to take more than a swallow or two in the beginning."

"I know. They talked with us about that already."

"Just expect it. After weeks of not being able to digest food, it will take a long time."

"I know. We'll try to be patient." I looked at the clock. We had talked more than five minutes. "Sorry, Marnix. I've kept you too long. You run. I'm going to watch D. try to eat."

"I wish I could see that," Marnix said wistfully.

AFTERNOON

"We're leaving," Boo Man's father told me in the cafeteria.

"Oh, that's great. What a big day for you!"

"That's for sure. The ambulance will be here to transfer him anytime."

"It's been a long haul for you and Boo Man. I'm going to miss seeing you all camped out across the hall, but I'm really happy for you. Really happy that he's gotten all the way to here."

"He's going to come a lot further. The rehabilitation place is going to be able to do so much with him. We visited them last week and saw what they can get these kids to do."

I stood up from my lunch to hug him goodbye. "You guys be good to yourselves and each other. I'm going to keep praying for Boo Man. You've been an inspiration to me not to hang it up when it gets hard."

He was very excited, very positive. "He's gonna make it. He's already starting to turn his head toward our voices."

I gave him thumbs-up and watched him walk enthusiastically back upstairs to his wife and damaged son. It had been three weeks since he snatched his baby out of their pool. He never left the hospital while Boo Man fought to defy the odds and stay alive. Now he celebrated the baby's emerging response to pain stimuli and contraction of pupils to light. As he departed for rehabilitation, no one could predict how much, if anything, Boo Man could recoup. But if there was any power in the force of determination, his father would will him back.

THURSDAY EVENING, APRIL 2

It had been an entire week since the last surgery and seven days since the last crisis. I submitted to the temptation to stay in bed a bit later, my body felt exhausted. When I joined Damion about eight o'clock, he seemed secretive and the nurses wouldn't let me into his cubicle until they finished doing something. When they did, Damion called excitedly, "Surprise! You can open your eyes now, Mom. Happy Birthday!"

Red, yellow, and blue balloons were anchored to the corners of the bed, and Damion was holding a gift.

"My birthday! I forgot! How did you all know?"

"We have our ways," Jane said, patting Damion's shoulder.

A larger balloon tethered to a coffee cup drifted over his head. Hershey Kisses and pink tissue paper filled the cup.

"Where did you get this? This is so wonderful!" The cup had an inscription: To the best mom in the world.

"I went down to the gift shop this morning," he proudly said.

"What?" I looked at my son and felt happiness spread over me. "That makes it an even better present!"

"They took me down in a wheelchair, and we picked it out."

"How did you know I'm a Kisses addict?" I asked the nurses.

"He said your two weaknesses are coffee and chocolate. This takes care of both."

"Oh, D. Thank you, everybody. Thank you, Damion. This is the best present I can remember. You all really surprised me. I had forgotten that today was even my birthday."

The nurses drifted back to work.

"This was really nice, D. It's a special, special cup to me."

"They helped me buy it because I don't have my own money with me."

"That was sweet of them. But you put in a lot of your own work going down to get this, button. Just the thought of that makes this the best present ever."

AFTERNOON

Baby Marty was going home. The cumbersome task of moving Marty began. There were all sorts of maneuvers made by nurses and the paramedics who'd be taking him home. The respirator and hoses were untangled and readied.

"Wait a minute!" M.T. interrupted. She gestured to Damion. "Marty, look who's finally gotten up to meet you and to wish you farewell. Come on over, Damion."

We rolled Damion's wheelchair up to the gurney, and Damion held Marty's hand. "Good luck, Marty," he smiled. Marty looked back wide-eyed.

"Good bye, baby Marty," I whispered.

"Marty's cool," Damion said as Marty and his entourage left.

FRIDAY, APRIL 3

As Damion benefited from his treatments and the passage of time, his chest x-rays began clearing. This did not permit us to slack off on therapy, though. Damion's lung volume still had a long way to go.

AFTERNOON

Damion had visitors today. We were surprised to see his Scout leader, John Holan. John brought his wife and his son Butch along. They were very nice, extremely nice to come hours out of their way. John handed Damion a plaid Webeloes scarf and a slide used to clamp it around the neck in the formal Boy Scout attire. It was the neckerchief for Damion's next age group in the Scouts.

They sat and spoke softly with him. I was so grateful they that they were spared the gruesome sight of seeing Damion before. Now all they confronted was a diminished version of Damion, a few tubes in place, winded when he spoke, and sipping on a concentrated drink with a straw. I could see their relief that Damion was looking better than what the reports in Dothan denoted.

But John felt horrible still. I could see it in his eyes and by the way his beefy frame cringed into our room. Before they left, I walked beside him in the hallway. "John, I've learned a little about how this happened since I called you. It's information that supports what I tried to tell you, that Damion's disease is not your fault. This disease results from contaminated meat. You couldn't have prevented something like this. It's like Russian Roulette: no one can say when the gun's going to fire."

"What about if I had made sure everyone's burger was cooked really well done?"

"John, how would you or I have known that? Show me one place where we've read or seen a public service announcement or a label or one news report that meat can now be tainted with a deadly bacteria and needs to be cooked differently than when you and I were growing up. The are no government or industry warnings yet, at least not in America, and some other countries as well. Besides, this bacterium has such an extremely low infectious dose. Something like salmonella takes millions of organisms to make a person sick; E. coli takes as few as one to kill. Moreover, there are lots of ways to get infected: handling the meat, meat juices dripping onto other groceries, and contaminated surfaces. People can't be expected to defuse an explosive substance like this in their kitchens, much less the woods, even if they're warned about it."

EVENING

"Bayne! Bayneroo! What are you doing here?"

My younger son was here! Right here in the middle of the hallway as I walked off the elevator. At first he tried to dodge out of sight, but there was nowhere to hide. Now he just came lumbering to me with a laughing, guilty delight.

"We were going to surprise you."

"Well, you certainly did that!" I kissed him. He was as darling as I remembered, still round and squeezable at eight years old. The baby fat on his cheeks was resilient against my nose. "Bayne, how could you be so sneaky? And how could you get here? Did you come down in a boat?"

He giggled like a conspirator. "No."

"Did you come in a car?"

He shook his head and when he did, his blond bowl haircut whirled a split second slower than the speed of his face. "Dad and I flew down in an airplane."

"You did! Oh my goodness! Well, that explains it!" I exaggerated my reaction to this revelation. "Just for that, I'm hugging you all weekend. Where's Papa? Is he sneaking around another hallway or what?"

"He's by Damion."

"Oh good. You want to come in with me? You've already seen D., too?"

"Yup."

"I bet he fell off the bed when he saw you."

"No, he knew about it. Dad told him on the phone last night."

"What! Don't tell me, Bayne! All of you are so conniving."

"Dad bought you a present from David Ethridge's store," he disclosed.

"Ooh, don't tell me, Bayne. Some things you've got to be sneaky about."

He followed me into the unit. There we found Marnix with Damion.

MIDNIGHT

After we put Bayne to bed, Marnix and I sat up beside Damion as he slept. Marnix wanted to get as much time with him as possible because tomorrow he'd leave again. I wrote a letter and he read. Sara tended to her charting. Dr. Rosenberg was back for the night behind his books at the desk. Everything was peaceful in the unit.

Then it happened again. An alarm on one of the P.I.C.U.'s monitors went off in another glass space. Instantaneously, its counterpart echoed from its associated monitor in front of Dr. Rosenberg. A nurse investigated calmly; false alarms were frequent and were disarmed simply by resetting the switches. But this one was persistent; despite the nurse's efforts, it cried shrilly for more attention. It came from the monitor next door, crying for the baby who could not cry. Now Dr. Rosenberg quickly rose from his station. The other nurses moved in, joined by Sara. Voices were raised. Then came the dreaded announcement over the loudspeakers: "Code nineteen, P.I.C.U. Code nineteen, P.I.C.U." Sara slipped her hand into our space, twisted the miniblind closed, and slid the glass door shut.

"Oh no," I said to Marnix. "Thank God Damion can sleep through this. Come on, little baby. Please don't die."

"It could be us," he said somberly.

Both of us sat and listened and waited. We heard the men in black rush in and the rolling of the crash cart. Then we listened to a long period of suspended quiet when voices were muted and time scraped slowly by.

Eventually there were sounds of people leaving and Dr. Rosenberg's voice at the desk. "Please call the mother and have her come in." I could hear in his subdued voice how sad he was.

Sara reentered our space and picked up her work where she left off. She had tears in her eyes. "What a shame, what a terrible shame that the tiny baby lost her valiant fight. We were starting to believe she was going to pull through. She was twenty-one days old today." Then Sara clamped her lips together as I'd seen her do whenever she felt strongly. She mounted her stool and sniffled as she resumed her paperwork.

Marnix and I sat there feeling awkward about leaving. A half hour later, Marnix tapped me on the knee and motioned for me to come from under the earphones. "I'm really beat," he said. "Do you think we can leave now?"

I nodded, "Yes, let's go. Good night, Sara. So sorry about tonight." I touched her shoulder. "Thank you for watching over D. for us."

We thought we were leaving the sorrow behind, but the sounds of a mother crying kept us from falling asleep. Over Bayne's breathing in the dark between us, I said, "You know what?"

Marnix grunted.

"I'm starting to feel like a veteran here. I've seen deaths, a drowning victim, disease, anarchy, abuse and all kinds of grief over these last five weeks. I keep discovering how precious our lives are for the short while we have them."

"Mmmm," he agreed, too tired to be articulate.

"I'm learning how wrong it is to waste our lives. But the biggest human evil has got to be callous neglect of the lives that depend on us. Look at baby Jimmy. And supposedly inspected meat almost killing Damion."

Marnix's regular breathing now joined Bayne's. The hallway outside our door was soundless: the dead baby' mother was gone now. The only sounds were the breathing of two of the precious people whom I loved, still safe within life's boundary.

SUNDAY MORNING, APRIL 5

Robert hadn't forgotten, nor had Damion. Robert came in as he had promised nearly a week before. His playful mournful expression was all-suffering as he made good on Damion's I.O.U. He said, "One word, Damion. Just one word. Luck. L-U-C-K."

"No, no, Robert. Talent. T-A-L-E-N-T," Damion laughed.

"They're dust tomorrow," the unquenchable Robert pronounced as he passed Damion his medicated hose. "Put this in your mouth and hush up. Tomorrow night in the finals they are dust. Michigan will put them out of their misery. Dust, Damion. They are going to die."

Damion couldn't answer with the tube in his mouth. He just listened to Robert with a Cheshire cat grin on his face.

As he manipulated the hose, Robert pretended to be all the more inflamed. "You just watch those finals tomorrow night," he teased. "They are going to die!"

AFTERNOON

A couple of hours before I needed to take Marnix and Bayne to the airport, Dr. Sastry came and sat in Damion's space and gave us the good news that we didn't dare dream about until now.

"Okay. We're set. The nurses will be moving you now. They are finding a room on the floor."

We were dumbstruck with a mixture of joy and dread.

"You mean today? You mean he's getting out of the unit today and going into a regular room?"

Damion was listening intently.

"Yes, it's time. He's ready. He can start physiotherapy tomorrow and of course he'll continue respiratory treatments."

No one said anything until Dr. Sastry left.

"I can't believe it," I said, too fearful to rejoice outright. I remembered all too well from the other hospital that being out on the floor meant diminished attention and concern.

Marnix asked me to come out into the hall with him. Out of Damion's earshot, he expressed his own concerns.

We were both so battered that we couldn't accept that the worst was over.

"I hope this isn't premature," he said. "There could be another hit. Oh God, I hope not. He'll be off the monitor. He won't have his own nurse looking after him. There won't be the intensity of care that he gets here."

We stood in the hall holding hands. Myriads of thoughts and fears unexpressed or half expressed cascaded through our minds.

Marnix wasn't a doctor now. Neither training nor knowledge counted. Our child was moving out of his safety net, our safety net, of vigilant care. He was going to the regular hospital despite the fact that he was still losing weight and there was no proof that his intestines were healed. He couldn't talk without his nostrils flaring, and he could barely stand without support. We were going to be on our own. There wouldn't be a monitor to signal another disaster striking.

I stood there wiping my eyes.

"It's final," Marnix said. "It's time for you to start clearing out his things."

"Are you crying?" Bayne asked when we entered the parent room. "Why are you crying?"

"It's nothing, Bayne. It's just that something I've looked forward to for a long time is happening so fast, and I'm afraid."

21

Standing

When Danny visited Damion's new room early the next morning, I told him how frightened I felt that Damion was out of the safety net of the unit's protection. "We still feel so reliant on you and the P.I.C.U. The nurses here are very nice and conscientious, but we're so worried that until he's able to eat real food and get a clean bill of health on his lungs, it's dangerous here."

Danny was understanding. He'd seen parents react this way before. "I think that you and Marnix have been battered by so many crises that you may be shell-shocked by now. It's hard for you to trust that Damion's gotten to the point of recuperation."

"But look at him, Danny. He's so weak. He can barely wobble to the bathroom. He just looks so fragile to us."

"I understand. That's why we've got work to do, starting today. I've lined up a physical therapist to work with Damion. First we'll get him to stand upright, then walk, a little more each day. He has to begin to use his muscles again. We'll do a chest x-ray and abdominal tests this morning. Dr. Kiros will talk with you about beginning Damion on a drink called Vivenex that will tide him over until he increases his calorie intake. And I'm still directing his care. I'll be seeing him a few times each day."

"Will you allow me one dumb question?"

"What's that?"

"If he gets in trouble again, will you take him back in a hurry?"

He smiled. "Of course, but let us do better than that. Let's keep him out of more trouble."

Before he went in to see Damion, Danny told me that he was the presenting speaker at a medical program on Wednesday morning in the hospital's conference room. It would be attended by pediatricians and other specialists on staff at St. Joseph's. "I'd like to present his case because it was a very complex and dramatic situation. Would you mind?"

"Not if it educates other physicians about H.U.S. and what it took for you to pull Damion through."

LATE AFTERNOON

We called Marnix from the phone on Damion's bedside table. Damion was upbeat and energetic so I let him do the talking first. He seemed to be taking the move to the floor more easily than I initially did. He saw it as the clear sign of progress it was. For Damion it meant more freedom, less intervention, more privacy and a whole new world to venture out into when he would be able to get around on "the floor."

"Hi, Dad. It's me, Damion. Yes, really. There's a phone on a stand by my bed. Mom told me I could call you and tell you what happened today. I did a lot of stuff.

"Well, first I went down to Radiology. No, in a wheelchair. It took a long time because first I had a chest and an abdominal x-ray. Then, later, Dr. Kiros gave me a special kind of drink until I can eat because today I could only eat some cream of wheat and drink apple juice. It's this powder junk that we mix up with different fruit juices, and it is awful!

"The fun part is that I get to go down the hall to physical therapy. They have all these floor cushions and giant balls that I have to do things on. The lady says my spine is crunched over like an old man's. First I have to learn how to stand up the right way again."

As Damion talked on, I studied the continuous scar knitting his chest and abdominal surgeries back together. Could it account for his stooped posture? Could it explain the drawing of his strength and muscles inward? It was a dramatic scar that might account for much of Damion caving in on himself.

I couldn't look at this scar without being struck by its heavy irony. This was the same incision used to eviscerate a beef carcass! This was the same cut made on the same cow that harbored the same O157 bacterium and whose intestinal contents splattered onto its sterile meat and created a vehicle for the deadly pathogen to infect Damion.

Who could look at Damion's scar and escape its circular irony? *So, now we are butchering kids.*

When I finally got on the phone with Marnix I gave him the good news about the reports that finally showed a normal-sized heart and clear lungs.

"This is great," he said joyously. "And the diarrhea has totally stopped. Now it's time to push that Vivenex, no matter how much he hates it or how putrid it tastes to him. It's time to get his G.I. tract operational again. It'll be slow but he's got to learn to eat and digest food again before he loses any more body mass. What's he weigh today?"

"One hundred and one pounds," I answered. "The last time we weighed him at home he was one-twenty-eight. That's a twenty percent body weight loss, which is extreme when you consider he was already a skinny kid before this happened."

"You're not saying this in front of him, are you?"

"No, of course not. He's been in the bathroom since he finished talking to you. He can make it there by himself now if he holds onto something like the bed or the wall on the way."

"Good. He doesn't need to hear anything so discouraging. Just keep it all positive. Because there are some tough things ahead of him still."

NIGHT

Damion was so tired from his active first day out of intensive care that he could only stay awake for the first half hour of the NCAA Final between Duke and Michigan. By half-time he was sound asleep. I took his glasses off but let him sleep in his hat. I kept the game on, just to be certain he wouldn't sleep through any miracle plays. Then at the end of the game when the nets came down and the plaque was presented to Duke, I turned off the television and went to the nursing station and asked if they thought it would help if I slept in Damion's room. They were different nurses from those on the floor last night.

"You don't have to," the nurse who was there said. "We'll be in and out all night to check on him. Get a good night's sleep in your own room. We'll keep careful watch over him."

"Thank you. Can I trouble you for some tape? Surgical will be fine. Thanks."

Damion still slept deeply under his magic hat. I made a sign and taped it over the screen of his television. It would be the first thing he saw when he woke up. I used a red and a black marker to make the large letters stand out. It said, "DUKE: 71 MICHIGAN: 51. Duke AND Damion are CHAMPIONS!"

The Duke players and Coach Mike Krzyzewski were an inspirational national championship team. I couldn't imagine them inspiring anyone more than one little kid in a hospital in Florida who fought alongside them.

TUESDAY, MARCH 7

Danny pulled the final lifeline this morning, the central venous line above Damion's heart. The TPN that had infused into it for thirty-four days was discontinued.

"That didn't hurt, did it?" Danny asked as he dropped the wire's tip into a sterile container to send for culturing.

"No." Damion's voice trembled with relief and gratitude. He was becoming less tolerant of needles and physical intrusions. This, too, was a good sign, I thought. It was not just that he'd had his share of pain and wanted it to stop. This renewed assertiveness had to do with coming out of his illness and establishing, "No. I'm not going to be hurt and poked anymore." It was a psychological component of his healing.

"So you know what this means, then?" Danny asked.

"What?" Damion watched as Danny stretched the last strip of tape on the gauze patch and threw its wrapper into the trash.

"It means that you are on your own. You're responsible for feeding your body enough protein and calories every day to get your strength and power back. Even if you don't feel like it, you've got to force yourself to drink the Vivenex and these Pediasure shakes."

Danny picked up an untouched Styrofoam cup filled with a strawberry flavor packet/Vivenex emulsion. He dipped his finger in and tasted it himself. "It's not so tasty, Damion. But what you need more than any other thing right now is to start to eat again. This will help you, if you'll just gulp it down."

"Okay." Damion took the cup, made a face, and swallowed four gulps as quickly as he could. Meanwhile I hopped up to grab a cup of water to chase it down, and handed it to him.

"Good boy. This will help to get you built back up again. Let's try to do this every hour or so, okay?"

"I'll try," Damion promised.

AFTERNOON

Sore and tired from yesterday's exertion in physical therapy, he tried without success to beg off when the therapist came to his room to collect him.

"Come on, we'll not push as hard today," the therapist promised. "We'll just do half and take it easy on the parts that really hurt. You know what they say, 'No pain, no gain.' Mom, why don't you come along so I can go over some of the stretching and exercise routines for when you go home."

Home? This was the first mention anyone had made about going home, and it startled me to hear it.

"He's going to need to be in an organized program for a period of time," the therapist said to me. "I'm sure you have a rehabilitation center within reach. You need to know what we're doing here to make sure there's continuity when you leave."

"Oh. Sure." I followed them out the room, the word "home" still reverberating in my mind.

When we returned forty minutes later, Damion saw a bag on his pillow. Climbing back in bed was more difficult than yesterday. After I stuffed pillows in the right places, I handed the sack to him. "This doesn't look like it came from Dothan or a cousin, D. It didn't come in the mail."

He reached inside and found a card. It read, "Glad you weren't in when I brought this by for you. I suppose you were out on the town celebrating. We'll discuss this later."

Damion was perplexed by this cryptic note. "Nobody signed this," he wondered as he reached into the paper bundle. Instead of scotch tape to seal the seams, surgical tape had been used, and the tissue paper was actually a padded white paper mat included in the sterile packs used in the hospital.

"Uh, oh. This looks like an inside job, Damion. Open it. The suspense is killing me."

Out fell a slip of paper with the words, "You were right." Then Damion unfolded an extra large T-shirt with Michigan across the back.

"Robert! This comes from Robert, Mom," he laughed.

WEDNESDAY MORNING, APRIL 8

The conference room was full for Danny's talk. Fifty or sixty physicians had settled at round tables after helping themselves to coffee and pastry. A sample of Damion's chest and abdominal x-rays hung on an illuminated board at the front of the room. Danny also had a slide projector and handouts. I fumbled through one at my place on the table. It started out with a brief description of Damion's admittance to St. Joseph's and then gave a history of his complications and treatment, including plasma exchange.

Before Danny began, he pointed us out at the back of the room and made generous remarks on how Marnix and I managed the ups and downs of the five weeks. Then he asked Damion if he'd like to tell anything from his perspective. Damion pulled himself out of his wheelchair and wobbled to Danny and the microphone. Although I had no suitable clothes for him down here, he looked resplendent at the podium in shorts and a T-shirt packed for Space Camp.

"H.U.S. was a very hard thing to go through. I felt terrible most of the time, especially when I had to be on the respirator a long time and couldn't drink. But I made a list of the important things that saved me so you can know what to do if any of your patients get H.U.S. Number one: God. Number two: Plasmapheresis. Number three: Danny and John Kelton who went to school with my dad. Thank you very much."

Damion got a hearty round of applause for his remarks. After he made it back to me and settled into the wheelchair, Danny politely let us know we could leave now by saying, "Damion since you've already lived through them, you don't have to stick around for all the boring details. Thank you for coming down."

As the door closed behind us, I heard Danny say to the doctors, "On this day of his pericardectomy, I gave him a seventy-five percent chance of . . ." And then his voice cut off. My whole body trembled as we walked away.

AFTERNOON

"How did your speech go?" Damion asked Danny.

"Just fine," Danny answered. "You did a good job on your part of the program."

I gave Danny my seat beside the bed and backed up against the window ledge that looked out onto the cream brick of the other hospital wings. This was their conversation so I just listened in.

"Damion, I see you have a birthday coming up on Saturday, and I have a proposition to make. What would you think if I let you out of the hospital early, and got you home in time for your birthday?"

"Do I have to come back after it?"

Danny smiled. "No, I mean for good. I wouldn't do this yet, except for the fact that you've been patient, I see you're trying hard to eat and get stronger, and also, I know that your dad can look after you as you finish getting better. Your mom and you have been here so long away from your family. Even though there is still a lot of work ahead for you, maybe you can do this in your own town in Alabama."

"We have a big rehab center in Dothan. My friend Matt's dad, Dr. Hall, is a bone doctor there. I could go work out on their machines and Dr. Hall could help me."

"Exactly. And I can call your pediatricians and explain where we are with you and suggest what I think you need in follow-up care."

Damion's eyes were wide with excitement now. "I can go home. That would be great. I can go home!"

"There are a few things I need before you leave. I want Dr. Brodsky to do another echocardiogram of your heart. And I want to see that you can keep down a few more things besides Vivenex and Pediasure. Something like scrambled eggs and oatmeal, okay?"

Damion nodded in agreement.

"And then your mom and I can talk about bringing you back here sometime in the future just to make the rounds with everyone."

Danny turned towards me. "He could get pediatric nephrology and cardiology follow-up in Alabama or he could come down in six months and let us look at how he's doing."

There was no decision as far as I could see it. "We'd rather come here. I'm sure there are excellent people in Alabama, but I'd rather have him see people who know his history," I answered without hesitation.

"That's fine. We can line that up when the time comes."

Dana, the child life specialist, was tapping on the door frame. "Hey, D., when you're finished, do you want to come help me on my computer?" Danny told Damion he could go now. After he left, Danny and I settled down for a wrap-up discussion.

"He's really happy; you can see that," I said. "Neither of us thought we'd be going home so soon. I suppose we've just become refugees here. We're going to miss everyone but it will be so great to go home and start over."

"I'm discharging him earlier than I normally would, but your husband can finish off what we'd do here. And if Damion stumbles, which I don't think he will, your medical community can handle him."

Danny faced me. "There are a couple things I want to discuss with you," he said. "First, how long it may take him to get back to all his previous activities and routines. John Kelton and I have talked about this. Our feeling is that you should both expect it taking six months to a year before his stamina, immune response and weight gain return. Some problems can go on for a long time. And sometimes these kids do well for a few years and then fall back into renal failure and high blood pressure later in adolescence."

"Yes." I nodded. "You need to be prepared for these possibilities and know what to look for. You need to expect that the immediate year ahead, maybe longer, could be a frustrating time as he recuperates slowly. He's been through a lot."

My enthusiasm was undaunted by what Danny was telling me. I couldn't conceive of what lay ahead. The only thing I could visualize was Damion getting stronger and steadily regaining strength.

But there was more to say. And this was the harder part that neither Danny nor I could dismiss. It was something I had spoken of only with Marnix during the urgent times when no one had a choice. It was a painful topic, one I preferred to examine sparingly. I said, "He's had a lot of blood. What about HIV testing now?"

Danny frowned. "He's had a lot of units. But I think it's a remote possibility. However, any possibility relating to this virus has to be taken seriously. You'll have to keep up the testing."

"I know," I said, downcast. Even to think about this was discouraging. I tried out the defense I had engineered. "You don't think it's possible that God would allow him to survive all these tough challenges of H.U.S. just to be cut down later by AIDS, do you?" This was a philosophical argument that I knew had nothing to do with the medical reality Danny was trying to get me to face. He didn't respond. So I asked him, "Well, how often and how long are you talking about?"

"No one knows for sure. There's no track record on this virus and infusion. H.I.V. surprises us all the time. Some recommendations are to test every six months for two years. You can talk to your pediatricians and Dr. Kelton and make your own decision based on their opinions."

"What would you do if you were us? If this were your son, how long would you worry?"

"If this were my son, I'd test for ten years."

"Ten years!"

NIGHT

I slowly walked to Damion's room. He wasn't there. I checked the teen lounge, the Child Life Office, and the physical therapy room. He was nowhere to be found. Finally, I checked with the nurses at the station. "Oh, he's with Andy in eleven."

"Who's Andy?" I asked.

"Andy's scheduled for orthopedic surgery tomorrow. He's kind of down so we asked Damion to visit and cheer him up since he's the same age and was looking a little bored himself."

I peeked in room eleven. "Hey, D. Hi, Andy." Both boys looked up but Andy didn't answer. He was a shy handsome child with black skin and a husky frame. He was immobilized in bed with the entire length of his leg in a cast. Damion sat in a chair pulled up to the bed. They were going through Andy's sports paraphernalia sent by our generous friends from home.

"Hi, Mom. I'll be there in a little while."

"No hurry."

For a few seconds I stood outside the door, my eyes filled with tears, and smiled.

Later, I asked Damion about Andy.

"He's scared. He's never been in a hospital before and tomorrow they have to saw his thigh bone. Do you think it was the right thing to give him my baseball card signed by Bo Jackson?"

"I think it was an outstanding thing to do. It will help him take his mind off tomorrow. He probably didn't expect to find a new friend here, D. It was good of you to visit him."

"I told him I'd sit with him when he comes back tomorrow."

"That would be a big help, D. You know how it feels to come out of surgery."

It made me happy to see Damion's maturing generosity and concern. I hoped all the goodness that came his way could reverberate to others. Evil leads to more evil. But goodness begets goodness. And therein, I have learned, lies the world's only hope.

22

The Ride Is Over

Thursday Morning, April 9

One final echocardiogram before Dr. Brodsky would release Damion. It took longer to perform and resulted in a longer report than all the others had. When all was balanced and evaluated, I saw a look of relief creep over the inexpressive face of Dr. Brodsky while he conducted each component of the comprehensive echo. The one important sentence of the report was its final evaluation: "This study shows no evidence of any residual pericardial effusion, and there are no signs of constrictive pericarditis."

"Dr. Brodsky, anything we need to do besides a follow-up cardiology examination and echo at six months?"

"No. We'll see how he looks then. In the meantime, I think he's come through this as well as anyone could have hoped for."

"Thank you for making that happen. We'll always be grateful that you were his doctor."

And then Dr. Brodsky did something he'd never done before, After all these weeks and all the travail of shepherding Damion through his repeated heart complications, he finally dropped his serious demeanor. Sidney Brodsky laughed.

Late Afternoon

Damion was resting in his bed. He was finally free of tubes and poles. Danny had pulled the lines out over the last two days, leaving only one IV capped off just in case he needed any medications before we left the next morning. Damion had had physical therapy, and kept his promise to check on Andy who was back from surgery. Now he rested contentedly as I came in and out to gather cards and gifts, adding them to the piles of our accumulation stacked on Marnix's bed. The mail room had given me boxes to pack our clothes and papers in, a job I'd finish up that night.

Dana rapped on his door. "D., why don't you come on with me? I need some advice on a new Nintendo game I just ordered for the teen room. Can you come give me a hand? I just loaded it." She helped pull him up; he reached for his Duke cap. Dana tied one sneaker while I tied the other. And we helped him up.

Dana looked at me and gestured for me to follow along with them. She placed her index finger against her lip to signal for me not to ask why. "And, Mom, why don't you come, too. I want to show you something that just came in," she said.

We moved slowly down the hall, Damion not rejecting my offer to hold one of his thin arms as he walked. Opening the teen lounge door, the room exploded with cries of, "SURPRISE!" Twenty or so people stood behind a long table covered with a table-cloth, plates, drinks, and a cake that said in blue icing, "Happy Birthday, Damion. We'll miss you!" It was incredible. Everyone was there: Danny, Dr. Sastry, Dr. Cahil and Dr. Kiros, all the P.I.C.U. nurses that were on at the time and some who weren't but came in anyway, Robert, and Pat from administration. So many of the remarkable people who did so much for us, who fought and struggled as a team to save him. They had taken a few minutes from their harried schedules to celebrate Damion's discharge.

Damion and I were amazed. We knew that every one of them had done their best to get us to this point. They were our friends, the best friends Damion would ever make. As we drank punch and talked about the last six weeks, I realized how hard it would be to leave them the next day. It would be impossible to ever forget this team of professionals who saved his life. We loved them all.

23

Home

I had the practical problem of getting the van home. Marnix and I talked about whether Damion was strong enough for a long car trip, or whether we should fly home and worry about the van later. But Danny said the car trip would be no more tiring than flying, and so we decided on it.

I pulled the van up to the curb lane with the security guard directing me. I loaded boxes and my suitcase in back and reached over the rear seat to put a bag on the bench. The towel, the kitchen pot, and the Emetrol bottle were there. I was astonished; how could I have not noticed them before? Had this stuff been there all this time like overlooked evidence from a crime? A six-week-old stain sunken in the pale upholstery made the nightmare real and graphic to me again. I saw vividly in my mind's eye Damion curled pale and lethargic in the back, his health just beginning to bleed away from him. I replaced the towel over the tragic spot where Damion must have hidden it. And then I watched him through the tinted rear windows. He was waiting at the curb in a wheelchair. So much had happened since this blood. So very, very much.

Ten or twelve friends waited beside him.

After we got him loaded and propped with pillows and strapped in the front reclining seat, I stood beside his open window. I had already hugged Danny and all the nurses in the unit who couldn't come down. "Well. What can we say?" Terri had tears in her eyes as she leaned in to hug him.

I turned to her, "Thank you, thank you, thank you for getting us through this. We're going to miss all of you."

A minute later as our van rolled away, they called:

"Goodbye!"

"Take care!"

"Be good, Damion."

"Stay out of hospitals!"

Glancing back at them all through the rearview mirror, I saw they didn't leave their positions until we had entered traffic and driven nearly out of sight.

Neither of us could speak until we were on Highway 75 going north. We were so choked up, reflecting on these people and how they helped us.

"D., do you know how exceptional those people are?" I asked.

He nodded his head in affirmation. "Some day I'm going to work in a place like that."

"Really?"

"Yep. First I'm going to Duke for medical school. And then I'm going to ask Danny if I can work under him so I can become a pediatric intensivist like him."

"You'd be a good doctor, knowing how it feels to be on the other side. But, Damion, whatever you end up doing, I think the most important thing is to come out of this mess wanting to help others like people helped you."

"Do you think I can come right after Duke?"

"Well, usually you have to do an internship for one year and then a residency for three, and then something like what you're talking about would maybe be a fellowship, or maybe a year of experience following a fellowship."

"Do you think Danny would let me?"

"I think he'd be very proud to see you helping children. And there's no one who could teach you more than Danny, that's for sure."

"Well, that's what I'm going to do," Damion said definitively.

After a few minutes, I remembered what my dad had told me when I took Damion as a three-month-old to meet his grandparents. Marnix and I had picked his name strictly on the basis of sound. But my father who loves history questioned, "Did you name him after Damian and Cosmas?"

"I don't know who they are."

"Third century brothers who practiced medicine without charging for their services. They're the patron saints of physicians and surgeons."

I didn't tell this to Damion now. If he could just stay healthy, there would be a lot of years and a lot of decisions between now and his career. I didn't want him ever to feel constricted by a name, or by any parental expectations.

"Do you really think Danny might say yes?"

I paused and glanced over at my son for just an instant. "D., I think if you work hard enough and want something badly enough, if it's really what you want, any dream you have can come true." Hearing my optimistic words flow so naturally from my mouth, I came to an important realization. Though the blind faith I had once had was now gone, though I had come to know and realize the presence of evil in the world, I still believed in the future, the endless realm of possibilities for Damion, for us all.

AFTERNOON

Damion stayed close beside me in the front seat the entire seven hours home. We talked about the feeling of exhilaration we shared. Going home meant lots of new plans: rebuilding his health, seeing his friends again, possibly starting school in a few weeks for half a day.

I watched the highway speed by as Damion dozed off. Trees that were bare when we drove down had now burst into full-blown leaf. The strong April sun traced Damion's chiseled profile, deepened by starvation. The wind rushing in through his cracked window ruffled the pillow case wedged between the seat belt and his wired chest. Time and the renewed landscape sailed by.

I could not help wondering if I had dreamed this before. There was a familiarity that seemed impossible. I told myself there's never been this trip with this child beside me, stripped of almost everything, reduced to this, sun and hope and gratitude streaming in the windshield while he slept. Yet somehow it was all jarringly familiar. The sense of déjà vu was so strong. Maybe, I thought, I'm mistaking this strange sensation for something once lived. Nevertheless, if Damion came out of this terror forged by a mission of helping others, what would my own purpose, still undefined, be? What was the point of his brush with death? Why was it our child? How would this change our lives? How would Marnix and I fulfill our responsibility, now that we'd been given Damion's life back?

The mysterious and the familiar teased and danced: they shimmered ahead in the illusion of water on hot pavement. They accompanied us all the way home. A hundred yards ahead always slightly out of reach, evaporating in the breezy air before our tires reached them. But as I drove on, a poem of gratitude seemed almost to compose itself:

Shining flag of a boy!
No longer tethered to the winter wires, anchored by taut whispers
Or grasped by the gloved hands that held you to this life.
See, your freedom has waited for you!

Resilient streamer of a boy!
Lift threadbare and thin, the sky a perfect azure hope
No tears to cry for your tattered boyhood.
See, your childhood has waited for you!

Rescued banner of a boy!
No poisoned winds to rip you, the cutting wires are undone.
Unfurl into the defiant Spring.
See, the Spring has waited for you!

Victory flag of a boy!
Strengthen while we hoist you aloft, fly unfettered and new
Back into your beautiful Life.
See, your life has waited for you!

Epilogue

FIRST THERE WERE HOURS. There was that wonderful homecoming moment when Damion wobbled across our kitchen, nostrils flaring wildly. There was that first happy evening settling him on a mattress beside Marnix's and my bed, pillows propped between his bony limbs. Hours went by, no emergencies occurred, he slept beside us, and our joy increased.

Then there were days. Days of unexplained fevers, days of abdominal pain, days of medical tests and lab results. There were nights of Marnix and I listening to him breathe in the dark, whisperings of thanks for Damion's life, rustlings of reverence no different from the awe he inspired twelve years earlier when we brought him home wrinkled and new from the hospital's nursery. More days went by and our reverence deepened.

Then there were weeks. Weeks of rehabilitation, deepening bone and muscle ache as Damion learned to stand erect and to regain full range of motion in his limbs. There were weeks before he could climb the stairs to sleep in his own room, and more weeks before he had the stamina to attend school all day. More weeks went by and his strength expanded.

Then there were months. There were months of flu-like illnesses before his immune system repaired itself. Months of relapses into breathing difficulties, a month when he was rehospitalized with pneumonia. There were months of learning new limits and boundaries, what Damion could and could not do. More frustrating months went by and his resilience grew.

Over time his broken body began to restore itself, and what it could not repair it learned to compensate for. Marnix and I came more and more to trust the hard-won peace that settled over our lives. Damion had ridden on a demonic roller coaster and survived because of heroic measures in surgery and therapy. Now he began to rebuild a functional life. As the months circled to become nearly a year, I believed more and more in his recuperation. Yes, it slowly became true. He emerged victorious from that deadly pathogen O157's vicious assault.

But our peace was incomplete. It became clearer to me that although my family had won our battle, larger wars lay ahead. Conflicts larger and more complex than I would ever imagine during that quiet year of Damion's recuperation.

While he healed, I read everything I could about O157. I started in the medical libraries and devoured the articles published on the disease and pathogen. My father's advice that etiology would lead to answers turned out to be prophetic. Etiology led directly to reports on previous outbreaks, to veterinary science articles, to the history of USDA's meat inspection program, to affidavits by whistle blowing federal meat inspectors, and to published regulations for the European Community. Soon I was talking with inspectors, investigative journalists, consumer groups, medical authorities, agency bureaucrats, microbiologists, meat scientists, and foreign public health officials. Yes, etiology led straight to policy. It led me to the disturbing realization that Damion's case was but a tiny skirmish in the larger onslaught of E. coli O157 throughout the world.

It was impossible for me to walk away from Damion's experience. It was impossible to walk away from the fight, not when the microbe's threat remained unresolved. I felt this burden whenever my car rolled up to a fast food window, whenever my grocery cart rolled past a meat case. Revulsion rolled over me whenever I came to the glistening red tubes of ground meat, whose origin I could only imagine and shudder! "These, Mom!" Damion once said to me in front of the meat case. "These! See, 'I.B.P.' is printed on the wrappers. Just like I remembered in my dream."

The frustration of the larger unfought war weighed most heavily as Marnix and I drifted off to sleep. My earlier belief in the system had evaporated. *Everything was not good. Everything did not work.* Not as long as a broken system let fecal contamination of food in so many countries put so many children at risk, not as long as so many parents knew nothing about this microbe's deadly threat.

The incidence of O157:H7 disease was rising dramatically. H.U.S., an obscure syndrome only a decade ago, had become the leading cause of kidney failure in U.S. children. In Argentina it was already a leading cause in pediatric death. Outbreaks unfolded in Japan, Germany, France, and Italy. In England, cases were linked to a huge fast-food chain. In South Africa an epidemic arose when infected cattle carcasses polluted a stream. Dutch children were stricken after swimming in a pond, and children on American farms were infected. In Canada and the United States, nursing home, day care center, and school outbreaks were sites of problems.

Modern transportation and relaxing trade barriers meant that within hours, infected food products could enter many countries. E. coli O157:H7 needs only one microbe to maim or kill, and its talent for cross contamination ignited outbreaks involving apple cider, mayonnaise, produce, even water. Because this microbe was colonizing the herds, because the food industry remained so laxly regulated, and because the public health network had little surveillance for foodborne disease, O157 became a smoldering threat, and at any moment in time, the start of a new and deadly nightmare could begin.

I asked John Kelton, "What can I do? How can we save other children? How can we help resolve the treatment issues? How can we get word on plasma exchange to people who desperately need it?"

"The treatment issues," John answered, "will resolve over time as part of the natural evolutionary process of medicine. If you want to save kids, focus your efforts on keeping them from getting infected in the first place. Do something to reduce the amount of contamination out there."

I asked some of the foremost E. coli O157:H7 experts at the Centers for Disease Control. They told me they had been battling *this demon* for years, investigating outbreaks and sounding alarms. No one appeared to be listening. What was needed was a grass-roots effort of affected people world wide to demand changes in the way meat is produced and inspected. They told me nothing would change until that occurred. "They've been waiting for us, Marnix," I told him that night. "They've been waiting for victims to figure it out, to stagger back up and fight."

Eleven months had passed since Damion want camping, yet the threat of E. coli was enlarging not diminishing. The threat of this emerging pathogen was like an evil apparatus whose springs were becoming more and more tightly wound, with the music of a demonic carnival ride playing on as the system cranked dangerously along. And then the metaphor came tragically and literally true. Exploded.

It started, for Americans, with a tiny spark that no one noticed. Little Lauren Rudolph ate a Jack-in-the-Box hamburger in San Diego, California. No one took a culture when she developed bloody diarrhea. When she suffered several heart attacks and her brain waves flattened, her mother was only told that Lauren died of complications of the flu. The local health department did nothing with her postmortem information concerning O157:H7 infection and H.U.S. diagnosis. Despite a cluster of H.U.S. cases and O157:H7 cultures in its jurisdiction at the time, the health department did not sound the alarm. Even if it had, California was not a reporting state and was not required to relay such an alarm to the Centers for Disease Control. America's tattered surveillance net failed miserably again. Tainted meat continued to be shipped to franchises of the Jack in the Box hamburger chain in several western states. In Seattle alone, nearly 600 tested positive for E. coli O157:H7 infection, scores of children were severely damaged by H.U.S., and three deaths besides Lauren's were officially counted (although several more people would have other causes of death listed on their death certificates, subsequent to having tested positively for O157:H7 infection).

Worldwide, Jack-in-the-Box was the watershed event, an epidemic so large, so well investigated that finally O157:H7 was ripped from the obscurity of medical literature and splashed across national and international headlines. Now there were many parents connected by the shared experience of our children's disease, and for some, death.

My first impulse was to get lifesaving information into the hands of those new victims. Finding some of their names through media reports, I sent medical articles to their hospitals for parents and victims to share with their doctors. *U.S.A. Today* published my letter condemning deplorable conditions in meat plants and criticizing our antiquated inspection system. Once the children who'd become ill at Jack-in-the-Box had been discharged or buried, parents in America began to interconnect. Seattle families organized a town meeting to explore the same questions with which I had wrestled. Some of the families were being overwhelmed by the crisis management exerted by both the meat trade associations and the USDA. Outrageous things occurred like trade association representatives cornering people in hospital corridors. Intimidating things like agency officials trying to divide and defuse parents in exhaustive meetings before they had an opportunity to voice their anger at public hearings. Dismissive things like the administrator describing parental grief and questions by parents as "forces of hysteria." I assured him parents were in no way acting hysterically; they were responsibly and logically asking the very questions that I had asked when Damion became severely ill. Questions like: *How could this have happened? What's wrong with the inspection system that a lethal bacteria does not violate its standards? What's to prevent this from happening to other children? Why were we never warned about O157:H7 when there were so many previous outbreaks?*

Parents invited me to speak at their meeting. "Marnix, I feel it is very important for me to go to Seattle," I explained, "even though I'll have to leave you and the children. I don't know what will come of it, but I can't sit by and watch what's happening. You've read all the media reports saddling the entire blame on the restaurants for undercooking the meat. And here, just read how the USDA minimizes the death toll since 1982, claiming only *'several children have died.'* Several! My opinion is they're either ignorant, or lying, or both."

Damion and I began to speak to the media and, most important, forged the beginnings of relationships that would grow into a national movement. Soon parents across my own country coalesced into what would become the first national organization devoted to eradicating bacterial food borne illness. S.T.O.P.: Safe Tables Our Priority. S.T.O.P.'s efforts to change the system were already too late for our own children. Our only agenda was to spare other families the same near tragedy that contaminated food inflicted on our lives.

In America the new Secretary of Agriculture, Mike Espy, was sworn in just as news of the epidemic was breaking. He said meat inspection reform would be USDA's "highest priority." But before the fight was over he, too, would become one of the war's casualties. Secretary Espy tried. He immediately hired several hundred new inspectors which helped to fill some of the more than 500 vacancies created during the deregulative 1980s. He promised the introduction of a science-based system which would target microbial contamination, the first system update since Upton Sinclair wrote *The Jungle* at the turn of the century decrying the horrifying conditions in the slaughterhouses of America.

Secretary Espy was well-intentioned but he was confounded by flawed agency architecture. Meat inspection fell under a USDA department entitled Marketing and Inspection, two conflicting functions under one roof. Policy had been dictated by the economic interests of the industry rather than the needs of public health. Espy's hands were also tied by holdover bureaucrats. The Food Safety and Inspection Service, FSIS, was directed by animal health experts and meat scientists whose expertise lay in disciplines unrelated to microbiology and public health. Their lack of public health comprehension was reflected in the agency's relaxed standards over the last decade. To me, it was revealed in their erroneous written description of H.U.S. as a mere "urinary tract infection." My moment of revelation came while sitting in a wing backed chair in the receiving area of the Secretary of Agriculture's office, waiting for an appointment with Mike Espy. An important undersecretary sat down to keep me company. He attempted to make polite conversation. "I saw your son Damion on Dan Rather, Mrs. Heersink. Has he gotten over his bout of hemo . . . hemo . . . What's the name? That hemophilia urinary something syndrome?"

"They don't get it, Marnix," I said later, talking to my husband from a pay phone at National Airport. "They haven't got a clue! This is *their* pathogen, their disease. Despite all the media heat of Jack-in-the-Box, the agency directors don't even know the name of the disease." This official's ignorance was my personal call to arms.

But for most parents it was a larger transgression that galvanized their anger. In the aftermath of the epidemic, Secretary Espy imposed a policy called "zero tolerance," which meant that fecal smears had to be trimmed off carcasses. Within days this basic health requirement was undermined. We obtained an intra-agency memo that challenged Espy's definition of fecal contamination and then, amazingly, suggested that the FSIS administrator wanted a list of inspectors who were enforcing zero tolerance too strictly. Parents were outraged by the callousness of the memo. One typical parent asked, "Does zero mean zero, or what? How can these inspectors do their job when they are not only harassed by plant owners, but are threatened with reprisals from their own agency?" The undermining of zero tolerance was consistent with everything I'd been hearing from whistle blowing inspectors, that not only were their numbers reduced and their autonomy eviscerated by deregulation, but that when they did condemn meat, their decisions were increasingly overruled by agency hierarchy in Washington. For all FSIS's stumbling, for all its inadequacy in public health protection, we could almost forgive them. But to parents of injured or dead children, the zero tolerance memo was an unintentional but irrevocable declaration of war.

Now the real fighting began. Parents of E. coli victims found ourselves smack in the middle of the contentious battles on meat inspection. Congressional hearings and media exposés. Heated public meetings in cities around the country. A wrenching symposium in the Senate building organized by S.T.O.P. and other food safety groups. Protests at trade association conventions. Press conferences. An industry lawsuit to delay labeling. Another industry lawsuit to halt O157 testing. Investigations. Leaked documents that were delivered anonymously to our mailboxes. Being the subject of Freedom of Information Act requests. Countering industry misinformation. Criticizing state public health departments when they covered up outbreaks to protect local businesses. Attacking senators and congressmen when they bowed to industry lobbyists. Exposing the predeterminism and lack of credibility of industry's "science." Allying ourselves with independent researchers. Taking journalists across the ocean to examine other country's systems. Calling for mandatory state reporting laws. Publicizing the continuing sanitation violations in meat plants. Demanding name brand accountability and trace-back capability for meat products. Drawing attention to the unrelenting E. coli outbreaks both here and abroad since Jack-in-the-Box. The last three years have been contentious. There have been many battles.

And some profound victories. A revolution has begun. In the United States, public health now has a chair at a policy table once dominated by industry. A modernized system of inspection is promised to be phased in, one that will set sanitation standards and target pathogens for the first time. E. coli O157:H7 is the one bacteria USDA now classifies as an adulterant—meat known to be contaminated with it can no longer enter commerce. FSIS has begun a limited testing program for O157:H7. Many other outbreaks and new research have established that cooking alone is an ineffectual public health strategy against this microbe. Whereas at the time of the Jack in the Box outbreak only eleven states in America had O157:H7 reporting laws, two-and-a-half years later thirty-five states had them. Legislators who have tried to block reform on behalf of trade associations have been stung by a fierce public backlash. Food safety has become the one regulatory issue politicians don't dare touch, overtly. Even some trade publications have come to admit that our meat supply may not be as safe as once thought. The public is becoming increasingly aware. For example, shows such as the United States-based television news program *20/20* reported in late 1995 that E. coli O157:H7 is reaching epidemic proportions. New microbial tests detect O157:H7 more rapidly. Technological interventions like steam pasteurization promise a safer meat supply in the future.

Damion's own battle and victory over O157:H7 has evolved for me into a larger battle. Yet, in my own mind, I'll always remain the most unlikely of activists. I am a mother and wife caring for my family. Despite this I have now become a public person. I find myself being interviewed on radio and television shows, traveling to Europe talking about E. coli O157. Sometimes I find myself giving a radio interview while nursing one of my squirming newborn sons, thinking of a sound bite for television while washing mud off Damion's soccer cleats, or composing Senate testimony on the back of a grocery list. The messages on our family's answering machine depict how truly odd my life has become. They reveal the vastness of the disconnect between the things I do each day (family) and the things I do each day (issue). There's nothing I want more than for the E. coli problem to be resolved.

Four long years have passed since Damion went camping. During these years we have fought a war, a war of words and ideologies, a war whose real casualties remain the tens of thousands of people who are infected, including the hundreds who die each year from O157:H7 in the United States alone while the grinding process of reform is snagged on political obstacles and industry delaying tactics. It has been a time of dizzying victories, a time of agonizing setbacks; but always, our commitment strengthens in the advance toward victory and a safer food supply.

Yet, every time I fax medical articles to desperate parents in intensive care units, every time another outbreak is detected in countries around the world, I realize the menacing threat of E. coli O157:H7 and other frightening menaces such as "mad cow disease" arising from our food supply being contaminated have not been eradicated. My mission will not be completed until our meat supply is safe and no more children die.

Afterword

By Carol Tucker Foreman,
Former Assistant Secretary of Agriculture for Food and Consumer Services,
U.S. Department of Agriculture;
Creator and Coordinator of the Safe Food Coalition

It never should have happened. Damion should never have been exposed to E. coli O157:H7, never suffered the horrors of Hemolytic Uremic Syndrome. But it did happen. It happened because the meat industry was more concerned with keeping costs down and profits high; because some members of congressional agriculture committees care more about campaign contributions from producers and processors than children at risk; because the United States Department of Agriculture, the federal agency responsible for inspecting the nation's meat and poultry supply, was staffed by people who came from and returned to the meat industry; because consumer activist groups concerned about food safety invested their resources in detecting minute quantities of a possible carcinogen than in stopping the approval of grossly contaminated meat; and it happened because the people of the United States say they want to reduce the size and influence of the federal government and vote for candidates who promise to get government off the backs of business, even if that business is a meat processor who is less than fastidious about cleaning old meat off the cutting board in his plant. In short, there is plenty of blame to go around.

Now we are on the road to addressing the problem of E. coli O157:H7 food poisoning. Many people deserve praise for having pushed government, the meat industry, the public health community and consumer advocates to this point. Mary Heersink and the other members of Safe Tables Our Priority (STOP) are first among those. They made it happen.

I first met Mary and Damion in Kansas City in a meeting room at a Lutheran Church where parents and friends of E. coli food poisoning victims had come to form STOP. They were joined by a crusading meat inspector and an attorney for whistle-blowing government employees. Also present was a reporter for the *Kansas City Star*. Three years earlier, he had written about school lunch and nursing home meat contaminated with what everyone described as a rare and exceptionally virulent from of bacterium, E. coli O157:H7, and about the children and elderly who died from food poisoning. He won the Pulitzer Prize for his series, but articles in a Midwestern newspaper didn't have much impact on Washington.

Mary and the other parents described the horrors of H.U.S. and the ghastly struggle of dying children who had done nothing more dangerous than consume that most ubiquitous American food, a hamburger. I met Diane and Michael Nole, whose two-year-old son had died in January 1993 after eating a fast food hamburger in Seattle. Michael knew I once had responsibility for the nation's meat and poultry inspection system and he asked me, "Lady, how could this happen? I took my kid for a hamburger and he died. The Agriculture Department people tell me it was because the meat wasn't cooked all the way through. How could I know that? I'm just a roofer. How could I know about E. coli O157:H7 and Hemolytic Uremic Syndrome?" Then he cried, and so did I.

Something important happened that weekend. These "victims" of a disease, an irresponsible industry, and unresponsive government started a revolution.

The STOP founders acted in the best American tradition. They saw a problem they couldn't affect as individuals, so they formed an association to educate themselves and to demand change. Like a mother lion cuffing an errant cub, STOP has called government and industry to account for their gross irresponsibility to this new bacterium and to bacterial food poisoning generally.

Mary Heersink's child almost died from a disease she had never heard of. Mary was determined to find out why, and when she did, she and her colleagues in STOP acted. They told the American people. They forced the Centers for Disease Control and the states to begin keeping records of H.U.S. cases and searching for and reporting the source of the food poisoning. They changed the almost hundred-year-old culture of the United States Department of Agriculture's meat inspection system, staved off industry efforts to maintain the status quo, and played a major role in stopping efforts of the new Republican majority in Congress to impose a moratorium on all health and safety regulation.

WHY DAMION GOT SICK

It never should have happened. The United States government and food industry officials brag that Americans enjoy the safest food in the world. The USDA spends over a half billion of the taxpayers' dollars and employs 7,500 people to examine all of the animals and birds slaughtered for food. It then examines meat and poultry products at each step of processing. For example, federal inspectors check cattle before they are killed, then examine the carcass. Inspectors are present when it is made into hot-dogs or lunch meat or mixed into a canned beef stew. Unlike other food products, meat and poultry processors enjoy the advantage of a federal stamp of approval. Check your supermarket counter. Every package of meat and poultry, except those packaged in the store, will have a seal that states, "Inspected and Passed—USDA" or "Inspected for Wholesomeness—USDA."

Despite these efforts, meats and poultry are not safe. E. coli O157:H7 is merely the most recent and dramatic manifestation of bacterial food poisoning that claims thousands of lives each year. The U.S. Centers for Disease Control and the USDA, estimate there are five million cases and 4,000 deaths each year attributable to contaminated meat and poultry. There are approximately 20,000 cases and 500 deaths each year from E. coli O157:H7. This is the pathogen described in 1993 as "rare." The USDA's Economic Research Service estimates that food-borne illness costs this nation about $2 to $4 billion annually in medical costs and lost productivity.

The CDC also reports that some types of food-borne illness are increasing. The increase may be traced to a number of factors, most of them influenced by late twentieth century American culture and demography. Today's food supply is highly processed, shipped across country, and increasingly, imported from other countries. Americans eat on the run, stopping at a fast-food restaurant, purchasing partially prepared or frozen food to be finished at home in a microwave. Each time meat and poultry are handled, there is an opportunity for pathogens to increase to a critical level or for clean food to come into contact with contaminated meat. When a food handler at home or in a restaurant touches contaminated meat and then grabs some carrots to chop them, the carrots become contaminated.

We are becoming more susceptible to food poisoning. We're an aging society and the number of people whose immune systems have been weakened by age or disease is increasing. Finally, as with E. coli O157:H7, new strains of pathogens continue to evolve, creating new challenges.

The nation's institutional arrangement for food inspection adds to the problem. Most food is inspected by the United States Food and Drug Administration. There is no question about FDA's assignment. It is located in the Department of Health and Human Services and staffed by experts in human health. Food and Drug Commissioner David Kessler is a medical doctor and lawyer, known as an ardent consumer and public health advocate.

Meat and poultry inspection is conducted by the United States Department of Agriculture. The USDA's primary responsibility is to promote the production and sale of agricultural products. However, Congress also assigned the Department responsibility for assuring the safety of meat and poultry products. That is akin to asking the Secretary of Agriculture to be both chief cheerleader for meat production and tough cop on the beat. It is hard to reconcile the conflicting roles.

It was especially unlikely that the secretaries appointed by Presidents Reagan and Bush would be tough cops on behalf of public health. Reagan's first secretary was a hog farmer. The next one was the former president of the meat industry's trade association. Bush named a cattle rancher and lawyer from Nebraska. But the USDA's conflict of interest problem didn't start with Reagan. The Department of Agriculture was created to serve America's farmers and ranchers, and consumer and public health concerns have always taken a back seat to advocacy for producers.

In the 1970's, President Jimmy Carter, a farmer himself, tried to change the ethos of meat and poultry inspection by creating an Assistant Secretary for Food and Consumer Services and putting that person in charge of meat and poultry inspection. The Reagan Administration believed inspection existed to serve the industry, so the inspection agency was moved to the assistant secretary responsible for marketing food products at home and abroad.

At the beginning of the Clinton administration, consumer advocates urged that inspection be returned to the consumer segment of the USDA and Secretary Mike Espy originally intended to do just that. It never happened, reportedly because industry leaders appealed to the White House to stop the change.

The leadership and staff of the inspection service has reflected its priorities. In 1993, the Food Safety and Inspection Service employed over three hundred veterinarians. It did not have even one medical doctor advising on how to prevent human health problems from meat and poultry. Under President Bush and during the first year of the Clinton administration, the administrator of the Food Safety and Inspection Service was a "meat scientist," trained not in food safety, but in the skill of breeding beef that tasted good.

The public has little patience with the boxes on an organization chart, but in government, where you stand depends on where you sit. From 1981 to 1994, the meat and poultry industry sat firmly in the driver's seat at FSIS.

The USDA's official policy with regard to bacterial contamination of fresh meat and poultry is a good example of industry's overwhelming influence on inspection. STOP parents asked the obvious question, "Why would USDA inspectors approve the sale of contaminated meat?" The answer was simple and shocking. According to USDA, meat contaminated with E. coli O157:H7 was not adulterated, and FSIS did not measure or limit harmful bacteria in raw meat and poultry.

In 1991, the head of FSIS told a poultry convention, "USDA does not now have the authority to impose microbiological criteria on raw meat and poultry." He went on to warn that, ". . . Congress, fed by misinformed public perceptions and pressured by misleading, so-called consumer activists, may direct us to do so." (Speech by Lester Crawford to the National Broiler Council, June 10, 1991)

On January 22, 1993, in the midst of the west coast E. coli O157:H7 outbreak, Russell Cross, administrator of the FSIS, sent a memorandum to Secretary Mike Espy stating, ". . . congress did not intend that inspection include microscopic examination." (Cross memorandum to Mike Espy, January 22, 1993, p.1)

Throughout the 1980's and into the Clinton Administration, the message from USDA was simple. Food poisoning bacteria are natural constituents of raw meat and poultry. Do not expect us to control them. If you cook meat and poultry until well done, you won't get sick. If you do get sick, it is your own fault.

The seeds of change were sown in 1985 when the National Academy of Sciences issued a report: Meat and Poultry Inspection: The Scientific Basis of the Nation's System. The NAS Committee provided the scientific rationale for a new inspection system that would concentrate on preventing health problems, especially bacterial food poisoning.

The report stirred some journalists and members of Congress to try to change the USDA's approach to inspection. Mike McGraw of the *Kansas City Star* and George Anthan of the *Des Moines Register*, told the story of archaic systems and toadying bureaucrats. Marian Burros of *The New York Times* covered the story regularly, and Bruce Ingersoll of *The Wall Street Journal* documented the story of the industry's influence. A few independent members of the Congress joined them. Neil Smith, a congressman from Des Moines and author of the 1967 inspection reform legislation, fought stubbornly to keep inspection honest. Senator Howard Metzenbaum introduced legislation to create a rational, independent structure for inspection. But most members of congress, especially those with the power to affect change, occupied their seats in part because they represented districts that produced cattle, hogs, and poultry and had no intention of offending the industry giants who kept the local economy strong and their own campaign offers full.

In late 1986, the Safe Food Coalition (SFC), was formed to coordinate the work of groups eager to see the NAS recommendation adopted. The Coalition's goal was to reform inspection along the lines recommended by the NAS. The group included: Government Accountability Project, Center for Science in the Public Interest, Consumer Federation of America, National Consumers League, Public Voice for Food and Health Policy, and United Food and Commercial Workers International Union. Consumers Union worked with the group as well. Today the Coalition also includes the American Association of Retired

Persons, American Public Health Association, Food and Allied Services Trades Department of the AFL-CIO, Environmental Information Center and, of course, STOP.

SFC was and is the loosest sort of organization, with no office, no by-laws, no dues, and no full-time staff. SFC began providing documentation of the problems in inspection and exposing the worst of the Department's offenses, but little changed, even after President Clinton's election and the west coast E. coli O157:H7 outbreaks.

Then Mary Heersink and her colleagues in STOP organized, and refused to be sidetracked or sweet-talked by the industry or government. Mary had researched E. coli illness and inspection methods in the United States as well as in some northern European countries. Her story was shocking and well documented. She was so persuasive that *Time* magazine sent a reporter with her to the Netherlands to report on the differences. Network news magazines picked up the story, and the STOP data. STOP established an office, hired a director and established an 800 number for victims to call for information and support.

The parents of H.U.S. victims came to Washington and told their stories. When the O157:H7 outbreaks kept happening, Washington D.C. finally took notice.

In August 1993, Vice President Gore's Reinventing Government team recommended that meat and poultry inspection be moved from USDA, to the nation's public health agency, the Food and Drug Administration (FDA).

The meat and poultry industry and its friends in Congress reacted quickly. Rather than lose complete control over inspection, they created a new office with the USDA, an Under Secretary for Food Safety. It was the first time in the Department's history, that meat and poultry inspection had been acknowledged by all to be a public health program. The Clinton Administration, which had been accused of being under undue influence by the poultry industry in the President's home state, set out to prove it could respond to both the health and political threats. Michael Taylor, deputy commissioner for policy of the Food and Drug Administration moved to Agriculture to become the administrator of FSIS and Acting Under Secretary for Food Safety. He brought with him Tom Billy, one of those talented, creative career civil servants who could redefine *bureaucrat* into a term of praise, and appointed the inspection agency's first medical doctor, Glenn Morris of the University of Maryland, who had served the NAS panel.

The new team at FSIS moved to reorient the message and the program. They began testing meat at packing houses and retail stores for E. coli O157:H7. Meat processors and retailers sued to stop the testing, but the courts upheld FSIS. After years of promises, FSIS published proposed regulations to institute a new inspection system, incorporating the Hazard Analysis and Critical Control Point (HACCP) concept, but also instituting microbial sampling and establishing performance standards for fresh and processed meat and poultry products.

When Republicans took control of the Congress in January 1995, many expected that Taylor would be driven from the Department and the industry would once again control decision making. They tried but failed. Dan Glickman, a former congressman from Kansas who had a long record of supporting food safety, succeeded Espy as Secretary and ordered Taylor to keep pushing reforms. In the Summer of 1995, meat and poultry interests attempted to sidetrack inspection reforms by attaching a legislative rider to the agency's appropriation. In years past, it would have worked.

But in 1995, things were different. The Administration vigorously opposed congressional effort; STOP members rallied and the news media reported their eloquent stories; and the Center for Science in the Public Interest (CSPI) appealed to its 700, 000 members to fight back. For the first time in history, the industry was split. IBP the nation's number one meat packer joined forces with consumers. Bob Peterson, president of IBP, argued that the meat industry was in jeopardy of losing its markets and urged Congress to keep HACCP on track. HACCP stayed on track and as this book goes to print, the USDA is ready to begin implementing its new inspection program.

The new approach to inspection will emphasize human health, require meat and poultry companies to take responsibility for assuring their products are clean, and require processors to test for microbial contaminants and establish performance standards that each plant must meet.

There will be more efforts by industry lobbyists to sidetrack the new inspection system and get rid of Mike Taylor and his team and the launch stealth attacks on effective inspection. House Republicans Pat Roberts of Kansas and Gunderson of Wisconsin have slipped an amendment onto the 1995 Farm Bill setting up an outside panel of meat and poultry scientists who have the power to review all FSIS regulations, including the new HACCP proposal, before they become final. The language was slipped in in a deal between the two Republicans and Senator Patrick Leahy of Vermont. It has the capacity to sink the new inspection program.

It isn't surprising to see this happen in an election year, when campaign contributions flow. But in an election year, the President and members of Congress are also susceptible to what the public wants. Mary Heersink and the members of STOP are an eloquent voice. They bring a moral authority that no one can argue with. At a meeting in the fall of 1995, a small meat processor told the Secretary of Agriculture that it was going to be very expensive for him to make the changes the USDA had proposed. He let the Secretary know that he had better ways to spend his money. Nancy Donley, a STOP member from Chicago, responded. "You're really just saying that it is inconvenient for you to make the change to assure your product isn't contaminated," she argued. "Well, let me tell you. It wasn't convenient for me to have my son die."

That is a hard argument to rebut. In the short run, the legislative sleight-of-hand will continue, but in the long term, inspection must serve public health and the inspection system must serve the larger public. People who fear that meat and poultry are dirty and the government inspection system corrupt, are likely to abandon both.

STOP and Mary Heersink offer a better solution for the public and for the meat and poultry producers and processors. Be responsible citizens.